Wilderness Medicine

FOURTH EDITION

by Wm. Forgey, M.D.

DR FORGEY is an Assistant Clinical Professor of Family Medicine, Indiana University School of Medicine, Northwest Indiana Campus.

He is also a Board Member and member of the Medical Advisory Board, International Association for Medical Assistance to Travelers, Toronto, Canada; Board Member and Treasurer, Wilderness Education Association, Saranac Lake, New York; Board Member and Editor, 1994 Position Papers for Pre-hospital Care of Wilderness Injuries, Wilderness Medical Society, Indianapolis, Indiana; Adjunct Faculty Member, Western Illinois University, College of Health, Physical Education & Recreation, Macomb, Illinois; and Adjunct Faculty Member, Slippery Rock University, Department of Parks & Recreation, Slippery Rock, PA.

ICS BOOKS, INC.
MERRILLVILLE, IN

This book is dedicated to my parents Gladys (Harmack) and Homer Forgey, without whose continuous love and assistance, none of this could have been possible. And to my brother Jonathan and his wife Florence, who round out the loving environment in which I was raised and in which I live.

WILDERNESS MEDICINE, 4TH EDITION

recycled paper

Printed in the U.S.A.
All ICS titles are printed on 50% recycled paper from pre-consumer waste. All sheets are processed without using acid.

Published by:
ICS BOOKS, Inc
1370 E. 86th Place
Merrillville, IN 46410
800-541-7323

Co Published in Canada by:
VANWELL PUBLISHING LTD.
1 Northrup Crescent
St Catharines, Ontario L2M 6P5
800-661-6136

Co-Published in Great Britain by:
CORDEE DISTRIBUTORS & PUBLISHERS
3a DeMontfort St.
Leicester, LE1 7HD
0533 543579

Library of Congress Cataloging-in-Publication Data

Forgey, William W., 1942–
    Wilderness medicine / by William W. Forgey. — 4th ed.
        p. cm.
    Includes biographical references and index.
    ISBN 0-934802-93-9 (acid-free paper)
    1. Backpacking injuries. 2. Hiking injuries. 3. Mountaineering injuries. 4. First aid in illness and injury. I. Title.
RC88.9.H55F67 1994
616.02'52—dc20   94-2004
                                                                              CIP

TABLE OF CONTENTS

Section 3
SOFT TISSUE CARE AND TRAUMA MANAGEMENT

Section 6
INFECTIOUS DISEASE

HOW TO USE THIS BOOK

There are four ways to rapidly identify which page contains the information which you need.

FIRST: A quick glance through the Table of Contents can lead you to the proper Section and Subject.

SECOND: The Primary Survey (pages 8–9) and the Secondary Survey (pages 9–14) not only describe how to perform a physical examination and what to look for, but it also refers you to the page of the book which tells you what to do about it!

THIRD: Throughout the book various sections have diagnostic tables with references to further evaluate or explain treatment options. For problems which fall into these categories, you can refer directly to these tables as indicated in the list below.

FOURTH: The CLINICAL REFERENCE INDEX, starting on page 231, provides a comprehensive cross reference between symptoms, conditions, and treatments. Subjects are listed using both medical jargon and vernacular descriptions.

PREPARATION FOR REMOTE WILDERNESS TRAVEL

THE PHYSICAL AND MENTAL ASPECTS

How do you tell a guy you hate his guts by the way he holds his fork?

Do not presume that medical problems will be the most significant challenges which you will encounter on a wilderness expedition. They are, frankly, leadership and expedition behavior issues. Any breakdown in this area can, and does, lead to the most significant of wilderness accidents—accidents which can easily magnify into serious medical disasters.

Most trips are not able to take into account the psychology and social skills of participants, but if this is possible it can avoid the stress and conflict that can make a dream project turn into a nightmare. I have found that a ten day preparatory trip is generally enough to identify idiosyncrasies that might indicate incompatibility.

The great outdoorsman Calvin Rutstrum once summed up this problem when he mentioned to me one day, "How do you tell a guy you hate his guts by the way he holds his fork?" It is simply amazing how personal habits and quirks can grate on you. In reviewing many successful (and not so) relationships during stressful trips, I have come to the conclusion that the most favorable relationship is one of "respect" - it surpasses love, hate, fear or any other human emotional form of interaction. If you truly respect a trip partner, you can tolerate mannerisms and faults that would otherwise be unacceptable.[1]

Plan a time schedule that allows for weather as well as terrain. Many accidents in the bush result from having to take chances while running out of time, food, etc., thus turning the expedition into a retreat, or worse, a retreat into a rout.[2]

Proper pre-trip physical conditioning cannot be stressed too highly. While trying to survive exposure, a major factor is the ability to generate heat, which is directly related to the ability to produce work. This is achieved through physical conditioning as the limiting factor, not by how much food one stuffs into one's face.

Obtain a pre-trip dental exam well in advance of the trip, thus allowing adequate time for possible needed corrections.

While a thorough physical examination is indicated for everyone, going to the extreme of cardiac stress testing (treadmill) is not required in persons without symptoms of chest pain. The exception would be the sedentary individual who was planning on significantly increasing the amount of exertion that he or she normally experienced.

Be certain that orthopedic deficiences, other impairments, and allergies are addressed in the medical history. Be capable of coping with the identified deficiencies by adjusting trip plans or personnel.

The pre-trip physical should include attention to immunization schedules that vary, depending upon the region of the world to be visited (see Appendix B). As a minimum, each trip member should have a current tetanus booster.

Make sure that everyone has had an eye examination within the previous three years. For those over forty, I recommend an eye exam (including glaucoma check) within the previous year. If significant vision impairment exists, carry spare glasses or contact lenses. Adequate eye protection, usually sunglasses, is a must for everyone.

Prepare an evacuation plan. Obtain adequate medical insurance, particularly if foreign travel is contemplated. And assemble a medical kit.

You're going to need some help.

The more that you read on this subject and the more medical training that trip members receive, the better off everyone will be. I recommend that you review the list of medical books in Appendix C. I particularly recommend that you obtain a copy of *Medicine for the Backcountry* by Buck Tilton and Frank Hubbell (see page 229 and Appendix C).

A frequent lament that I hear from prospective expedition members is not knowing a physician who could help by writing prescriptions for an adequate expedition medical kit. It is for this reason that the first edition of this book had an extensive non-prescription medical kit designed to handle most problems that one might encounter in the bush. A list of suppliers of the non-prescription medications and virtually all of the instruments and high-tech bandaging material described in this book can be obtained from the publisher by writing to: ICS Books, Inc., P. O. Box 10767, Merrillville, IN 46411-0767. I have personally tried to help each and every person writing me for advice in obtaining requisite medical supplies.

And prepare yourself mentally to enjoy the trip. Be expecting both adversity and monotony on any long expedition. A wonderful publication that shows the insight necessary for this to succeed is a little book by David Scott, *Paradise Creek*, due in the spring of '95 from ICS Books. I believe this book epitomizes what a long expedition is all about. As I helped prepare and sponsor David and his partner, Scott Power, for their expedition, you'll even learn a little about me in there, too.

THE WILDERNESS EXPEDITION MEDICAL KIT

The ideal medical kit will have multi-functional components to reduce the cost, bulk, weight, and simplify usage. It should also be modular to allow an increasing depth of care by including the more sophisticated modules only if the potential risks of the trip, or reduced access to medical help, warrants their inclusion.

Most injuries and conditions described in this book can be treated with very little in the way of kit components. But I have included here state-of-the-art items that would provide ideal treatment aid. As this book has been written for those who may be isolated without ready access to professional medical care, the treatments discussed go beyond normal first aid. The kit described in Appendix A similarly goes beyond what would be considered a "first aid" kit. But the initial modules are indeed easily useable under first aid conditions. The kit consists of six units: Topical Bandaging Module, Non-Rx Oral Medication Module, Orthopedic Module, Field Surgical Module, Rx Oral/Topical Medication Module, and the Rx Injectable Module.

As a minimum, the Topical Bandaging Module and Non-Rx Oral Medication Module will generally fulfill the vast majority of emergency treatment requirements. The Field Surgical Module and the prescription modules are designed for long term, and more advanced patient care. All items listed in the kit modules can be obtained without a prescription, except in the modules clearly marked "Rx."

In addition to the above, everyone should carry a new piece of emergency equipment called "The Extractor." This 4 oz plastic suction device is ideal for use in the first aid treatment of snake bite, puncture wounds, and venomous stings. It is far superior to the rubber suction cup snake bite kit. Note description of use on page 149.

Consideration must be given to a dental kit. Several are commercially available through backpacking and outdoor outfitters. As a minimum, a small bottle of oil of cloves can serve as a topical toothache treatment, see page 58.

A fever thermometer may be handy, but frankly, I never carry one. People wearing contact lenses should carry the special suction cup or rubber pincher device to aid in their removal. Consideration may be given to a stethoscope and blood pressure cuff, if you know how to use them. They are must items for Search and Rescue Units, but not for the usual wilderness expedition.

Early pregnancy detection kits may have a role in long term expeditions and in trekking or taking clients into wilderness areas. This kit is potentially useful when trying to determine the cause of severe lower abdominal pain in a female of child bearing age, the concern being the possibility of a tubal pregnancy which is a life-threatening emergency.

Provide an adequate means of water purification as indicated on page 71. Failing to do so can also be the cause of severe lower (and upper) abdominal pain. While I prefer the Katadyne water filtration system, water treatment can be as simple as bringing water to a boil.

Do I bring all of the items which I have listed in the Wilderness Medical Kit Modules in Appendix A? Yes! And no! It depends.

If hiking the Appalachian Trail I would carry a few pieces of Spenco 2nd Skin and tape, ibuprofen, Imodium, and possibly a decongestant. The rest of my load would be food and the other direct necessities of life, certainly not first aid items. For a three week canoe trip in Northern Canada with three other people, I would cut the quantities of the Appendix A kit drastically, but I would have representative items from each module along. For two of us spending six months in an isolated cabin or on a yacht in the Pacific, I would carry the Appendix A modules as written. Going with a team of 130 assaulting a mountain, I'd add a lot more stuff. But the exact nature of that stuff would depend upon my assessment of the situation. This book and Appendix A should give you a plan for the management of most remote area emergencies.

Occasionally, use of items brought along for various other purposes is made for medical reasons. From the cook, the medic needs to borrow baking soda, salt, and sugar in the management of profound diarrhea. The formula for making oral rehydration salt solution from these items is on page 70.

Vinegar, flour, and ammonia are useful in treating jellyfish tentacle attachments (page 158). Vinegar is also useful in treating sea urchin spine wounds (page 157) and sponge rash injuries (page 159). Cooking oil is useful in killing a bug stuck in an ear (page 52). It can also help treat dry lips and chafing.

Soap for cleaning wounds may also be obtained from the kitchen, if a surgical scrub is not carried in the medical kit. Granulated sugar sprinkled on abrasions is a field expedient method of preventing infection when there are no antibiotics available.

Each fishing kit should have wire cutters, possibly required to remove a hook from people, as well as fish. These wire cutters may also be used to destroy a zipper, sometimes a necessary project if someone has caught his skin in the zipper mechanism.

To prevent and treat hypothermic conditions, synthetic or wool clothing is needed, especially hat, socks and shirts. Having adequate sleeping bags, and choosing those that twin, may prove life-saving in hypothermic conditions. It is surprising how many bags will twin, sometimes the foot of one to the head of the other.

Matches are a potential lifesaver and should be available on every trip. I point out that a fire is a poor way of keeping warm; adequate clothing is the best solution for that problem. But building a giant fire is a method of getting warm in an emergency.

On extended trips a vitamin supplement might be in order to prevent deficiency medical syndromes, such as scurvy. There is no doubt that vitamin deficiencies ranked high among the reasons for death during the early days of polar exploration. We are not immune from them during the modern era either.

And for treating headaches, sometimes a cup of coffee is just the answer, especially if the victim is having caffeine withdrawal.

ASSESSMENT AND STABILIZATION

ASSESSMENT AND CARE

The aid of a victim of injury is similar to appropriate treatment of sickness or sudden complaint of pain from a non-injury cause in that proper care can only result if several basic steps are performed properly. The basics are straightforward. You should not be intimidated by this process. The problem with medicine in general is that there are so many possible diagnoses and treatments that the whole thing seems overwhelming. It is really not, however, if you follow certain logical steps.

These logical steps form the basis of starting the decision tree that will lead almost automatically to a correct course of action. They simplify the process into a much less scary proposition. The initial phase is assessment, then comes the treatment or stabilization phase. The first-aid approach would only include assessment, but this book is concerned with developing approaches to definitive treatment that could be reasonably performed in remote areas by relatively untrained (and undoubtedly very concerned) friends of the suddenly impaired.

Trauma assessment is divided into two phases commonly called the primary survey and secondary survey. What good is a survey if you don't know what to do with the information? During Search and Rescue operations what you do with the information is to record it. This recorded information, which includes the reassessment data, can be valuable to physicians at treatment centers as it indicates either a stable patient or a deteriorating one and helps direct their future course of action. For those of us who are stuck with caring for the patient in a remote area, this data can be used to enter a decision tree that will help determine our best course of action. Sometimes this will be definitive treatment, other times it will amount to minimizing the damage and striving to keeping the victim as functional as possible.

PRIMARY SURVEY

SURVEY THE SCENE

First: Before assessing the patient, assess the scene! Accidents tend to multiply. Make sure the scene is safe for the rescuers and the victim. Ensure that the situation does not become worse. This step can include such diverse aspects as avoiding further avalanche or rock falls to ensuring an adequate clothing and food supply for rescuers. Initially, however, scene assessment is to look for immediate hazards that might result in more casualties among the group attempting to help the victim.

AIRWAY

Second: Check the airway. If the victim can talk, his airway is functioning. In an unconscious patient, place your ear next to his nose/mouth and your hand on his chest and look, listen, and feel for air movement.

No air movement: check to see if the tongue is blocking the airway by pushing down on the forehead while lifting the chin. In case of possible neck injury, the airway can be opened with a lift of the jaw without movement of the neck.

Still no air movement: pinch his nose and seal your mouth over his and try to force air into his lungs.

Still no air movement: perform the Heimlich maneuver, see page 18.

Once you are able to establish air movement, continue until the victim can take over on his own, see page 22.

CIRCULATION

Check circulation by placing several of your finger tips lightly into the hollow below the angle of the patient's jaw.

No pulse: Start CPR, see page 20.

FIGURE 1.
Position of fingers to check for the carotid artery pulse.

SEVERE BLEEDING

Check quickly for severe blood loss. Check visually and with your hands. Slide your hand under the victim to ensure that blood is not leaking into the ground or snow and check inside bulky garments for hidden blood loss. *Severe bleeding*: Use direct pressure, see page 86.

CERVICAL SPINE

During the primary survey keep the head and neck as still as possible if there is any suspicion of a cervical spine injury. Suspicions should be high if the patient is unconscious or accidents such as falls from heights, sudden stops, or significant blows to the head. See treatment of cervical spine injuries, page 125.

Buck Tilton and Frank Hubbell in their excellent book *Medicine for the Backcountry* state "Do not let fear of spinal cord injury blind you to more immediate threats to life. If the scene is not safe, the patient may need to be carefully moved. If the airway is not open, grasp the sides of your patient's head firmly, and pull with steady, gentle traction and attempt to align the head and neck with the rest of the body. Gentle traction should be maintained until mechanical stabilization can be improvised (see spinal cord management on page 126)." [3]

SECONDARY SURVEY [4]

THE PHYSICAL EXAM

When the immediate threats to life have been controlled, our assessment needs to extend systematically over the entire patient, evaluating the extent of the known injuries, and looking for unsuspected damage hidden by the pain and the obvious. The situation will determine the sequence and thoroughness of this examination. But all patients deserve a complete, hands-on, head-to-toe check. In a small child, you may wish to go toe-to-head, gaining their confidence before attacking their vulnerable head and chest.

General guidelines for the patient exam include:

1. Gentle but firm palpation (feeling) of all relevant body parts, looking for obvious damage, pain responses, swelling, deformities, and abnormalities.

2. Moving the patient as little as possible, and not aggravating known injuries.

3. When necessary, cutting away clothing to visualize suspected injuries.

4. Communicating with the patient through the entire process, even if they appear unconscious. They are the questions, and they are the answers!

Specifically move from head to toe, Looking, Asking, and Feeling (LAF) for the signs and symptoms of problems.

HEAD: Look for damage, discoloration, and blood or fluid draining from ears, nose, and mouth. Ask about loss of consciousness, pain, or any abnormal sensations. Feel for lumps or other deformities.

Loss of consciousness, see page 11
Ear trauma, see page 53
Eye trauma, see page 35
Nose trauma, see page 47
Mouth trauma, see page 57

NECK: Look for obvious damage, or deviance in the trachea. Ask about pain and discomfort. Feel along the cervical spine for a pain response.

Cervical spine trauma, see page 125
Trachea trauma, see page 19

CHEST: Compress the ribs from both sides, as if squeezing a bird cage, keeping your hands wide to prevent the possibility of too much direct pressure on fractures. Look for damage or deformities. Ask about pain. Feel for instability.

Chest trauma, see page 143

ABDOMEN: With hands spread wide, press gently on the abdomen. Look for damage. Ask about pain and discomfort. Feel for rigidity, distention, or muscle spasms.

Abdominal pain, see page 62

BACK: Slide your hands under the patient, palpating as much of the spine as possible.

Spine trauma, see page 126

PELVIS: Cup the iliac crests with your hands, pressing gently down, and pulling toward the midline of the body. Ask about pain. Feel for instability.

Hip or pelvis pain, see page 138

LEGS: With your hands surrounding each leg, one at a time, run from the groin down to the toes, squeezing as you go. Note especially if there is a lack of circulation, sensation, or motion in the toes.

SHOULDERS AND ARMS: One at a time, with hands wide, squeeze each shoulder, and run down the arms to the fingers. Check for circulation, sensation, and motion in the fingers.

Orthopedic trauma, see page 128

A written or dictated note of all possible injuries should be kept. Don't let known injuries keep you from a thorough examination. Soon you will be treating all suspected damage.

THE VITAL SIGNS

An accurate measurement of a body's vital functions do not tell you what is wrong with your patient. But they do relate how well your patient is doing. The second set of vital signs is more important that the first set. And the third more important than the second. Circumstances will dictate how often the signs are taken, but the change over time is the key to using vital signs in long-term patient care. A constant monitoring of your patient should be maintained until they are "out of the woods."

LEVEL OF CONSCIOUSNESS: A normal level of consciousness allows your patient to answer intelligently in a way that tells you he or she is oriented in person, place, and time. They should know who they are, where they are, and generally what time it is. The level of consciousness is the easiest sign to assess, and the first to change. It can be recorded easily using the AVPU scale, which assigns the patient a letter grade from alert to unresponsive.

ALERT: The patient seems normal, and answers intelligently questions about person, place, and time. They know essentially what happened to them.

VERBAL: The patient is not alert, but they do respond in some way when spoken to.

PAIN: The patient does not react to verbal stimuli, but they do react to being pinched or rubbed in sensitive areas.

UNRESPONSIVE: The patient does not respond to stimuli.

PULSE: In the Primary Assessment you noticed a pulse at the carotid artery, assuring yourself your patient had blood being pumped to the brain. Now you are interested in the rate, rhythm, and quality of that pulse. Using the radial pulse, inside the wrist, where the thumb side of the hand joins the arm, is much more comfortable for the patient than pressing their neck. Press lightly with several fingertips.

RATE: The number of beats per minute. A range of 60-80 is normal in an adult. It will usually be higher in children, sometimes reaching a norm of 160 in an infant. Counting for one full minute is more accurate, but a count for 15 seconds and multiplying by four is acceptable and most often used. In the absence of a watch, take a pulse anyway. At least you can assess the rhythm and quality.

RHYTHM: There will be either a clock-like regularity, or a sporadic irregularity.

QUALITY: This refers to the force exerted by the heart on each beat. The force will be best judged by its relation to previous pulse checks. A Normal quality is strong, a Thready pulse is weak and an indication of inadequate circulation, and a Bounding pulse is abnormally forceful.

An absence of a radial pulse is cause for alarm. But delay panicking until you check the other arm. The cause might be an injury to the arm or shoulder.

Increasing pulse rate, see shock, page 16

Deformed fracture causing decreased pulse, see page 120

RESPIRATIONS: A patient alerted to the fact that you're checking their respirations may voluntary alter their breathing pattern. Keep your assessment a secret.

RATE: An adult normally breathes 12-18 times per minute. Children and infants breath faster.

RHYTHM: Normally, we breathe evenly and regularly, exhalations taking slightly longer than inhalations. Watch for shallowness or deepness, and irregularities in the pattern.

QUALITY: Normal breathing is quiet and effortless. Abnormal breathing might include labor, pain, noise (snores, squeaks, gurgles, gasps), and a flaring of the nostrils.

Respiratory difficulty, see page 18

SKIN: It's on the outside, away from the body's core where vital life processes are centered, but the skin gives pertinent information on the general well-being of our patient.

COLOR: Pink is the normal color of skin, pink in the non-pigmented areas of the body—the lining of the eye, inside the mouth, fingernail beds. It may be difficult to detect subtle changes in darker complexions, but the overall color of the skin is also an indicator. The size of the blood vessels near the skin determine color. Vasodilation (widening vessels) produces a red, flushed color, and indicates problems such as fever or hyperthermia. Vasoconstriction (narrowing vessels) produces pale or blotchy skin, and may indicate shock or hypothermia. A blue hue, called cyanosis, shows a lack of oxygen, and often indicates heart failure. Yellowish skin tells of liver failure.

Fever, see page 28
Hyperthermia, see page 188
Shock, see page 16
Hypothermia, see page 182
Yellow skin, see jaundice, page 168

TEMPERATURE: The temperature of the skin can be significantly lower than the body's core and still be perfectly healthy. It will indicate, though, whether the patient is vasodilating and growing warmer, or vasocontricting and getting cooler.

MOISTURE: Normal skin is relatively dry. Warmth and wetness from excessive sweating may be evident, but if the skin is cool and moist, it may indicate shock.

BLOOD PRESSURE: BP's are impossible to take without a device called a sphygmomanometer, and are more accurate if you have a stethoscope as well. It is mentioned briefly here because of its importance, along with a very crude field assessment technique.

Your beating heart creates pressure on the walls of your blood vessels. Without that pressure within the circulatory system, the oxygen-carbon dioxide transfer would not take place down on a cellular level. When the pressure drops too low for perfusion and adequate oxygenation to occur, tissues begin to die, and soon the organism follows. Blood pressure has two components: 1) the systolic pressure, measured when the heart is contracting, and 2) the diastolic pressure measured when the heart is at rest. A general norm is written as 120/80, but the pressure varies greatly from individual to individual.

As the pressure drops, skin becomes more and more cyanotic. Pulses begin to disappear. You'll lose the pulse in your feet first, then your wrist, and, finally, your neck. If you found the radial pulse of your patient earlier, and now it's gone, they are losing pressure. Prior to the blood pressure dropping, the heart attempts to compensate by increasing the pulse rate. If the pulse rate is increasing, try to correct the underlying cause. Sometimes this is due to fright (see page 23), high altitude injury (see page 196), fainting or vagal syncope (see page 26), anaphylaxis or severe allergic reaction (see page 145), or internal or external blood loss.

THE MEDICAL HISTORY

As you practice, you will gain pride in your ability to perform a patient exam and to take a set of vital signs. But the tricky part of assessment, and probably 80% of your final verdict, will come from the information gathered as you interview your patient.

Approach with a calm, confident attitude, whether you feel it or not. An aura of calmness surrounding the scene will often do more for the sick and injured than all the splints and aspirin you can throw at them. Quietly tell them your name and that you can help them. Don't scream, "What happened, What happened?"

If you haven't already, establish a relationship with your patient. It is more effective to say sincerely, "I know you must be afraid and in pain, but we'll make you as comfortable as possible," as opposed to panting, "You'll be OK, you'll be fine."

Create a positiveness about the situation. Say, "Are you more comfortable sitting up or lying down?" Don't say "Which hurts more?"

Be enthusiastic without being a cheerleader. Be kind without being nauseating. Be honest without saying everything you're thinking. Beware of the tone of your voice. Beware of your patient's tendency to take the slightest offhand comment as truth. Discuss with them the possible plans of action. They have a right to their say in what happens.

A helpful mnemonic is AMPLE:

ALLERGIES: "Are you allergic to anything you know of?" MEDICATIONS: "Taking anything currently?"

PAST HISTORY: "Is there anything possibly relevant I should know about your health?" Or, "Has anything like this happened before?"

LAST MEAL: "When did you eat or drink last?"

EVENTS: "What led up to this?" and finally "Is there anything else I should know?"

The questions you ask should not lead the patient on. Don't ask, "Is it a sharp pain?" Ask instead, "Can you describe the pain for me?"

If they are in pain or discomfort, another mnemonic is PQRST. What, if anything PROVOKES the pain? What is the QUALITY of the pain? Does it RADIATE? Describe the SEVERITY? And what TIME did the problem start?

If your patient is unconscious, you have to become even more of a Sherlock Holmes in your search for clues. Are they wearing Medical Alert tags on neck, wrists, ankles? Is there information in their pockets? What can you learn from witnesses? From anyone around who knows them? What evidence does the scene hold for you? Seek answers to the AEIOU TIPS: Is their unconsciousness the result of ALLERGIES, EPILEPSY, INFECTION, OVERDOSE, UNDER-DOSE, TRAUMA, INSULIN, PSYCHOLOGICAL disorder, or STROKE?

THE SOAP NOTE

When time allows, or if there are spare hands at the scene, all the information gathered during the assessment, and what was done for treatment, should be recorded on paper. You will never remember everything, vital signs slip away like autumn leaves in a high wind, and the patient deserves to have any physician who later takes over know the details of what happened and what was done. The note also becomes a legal record if a medicolegal question arises. Even if you're not sure what you're doing is absolutely correct, you want to record all your efforts in the patient's behalf. It shows you did your best.

The note can be divided into four sections for convenience or memory.

SUBJECTIVE: What happened to who (include age, address, and sex) where, and when? What is their chief complaint?

OBJECTIVE: What did the physical exam reveal? What are the vital signs, and when did you do the following checks? What is the relevant medical history?

ASSESSMENT: What are the possible problems?

PLAN: What are you going to do?

Eventually you'll add to the note your name and the names of any other members of the aiding party and witnesses.

As mentioned, the reassessment information is even more important that the first set of information taken during the initial secondary survey. How often the secondary survey needs to be repeated and how extensive it needs to be depends primarily on the history of the event. Very serious appearing events could initially require total body reassessment every 15 minutes. There can be no hard and fast rule concerning how often to repeat and how extensive the reassessments must be. There is no escaping the use of common sense. Eventually reassessment every few hours, even discontinuing this process will become proper. This is particularly appropriate when the examination is unchanged, stable, the patient is alert, and you have obviously effectively dealt with the injury(ies).

SHOCK

Shock is a deficiency in oxygen supply reaching the brain and other tissues as a result of decreased circulation. An important aspect of the correction of shock is to identify and treat the underlying cause. Shock can be caused by burns, electrocution, hypothermia, bites, stings, bleeding, fractures, pain, hyperthermia, high altitude cerebral edema, illness, rough handling, allergic reaction (anaphylaxis), damage or excitement to the central nervous system, dehydration from sweating, vomiting or diarrhea, or loss of adequate heart strength. Each of these underlying causes is discussed separately in this text.

Shock can progress through several stages before death results. The first phase is called the "compensatory stage" during which the body attempts to counter the damage by increasing its activity level. Arteries constrict and the pulse rate increases, thus maintaining the blood pressure. The next phase is called the "progressive stage" when suddenly the blood pressure drops and the patient becomes worse, often swiftly. When they have reached the "irreversible stage" vital organs have suffered from loss of oxygen so profoundly that death occurs even with aggressive treatment.

Consider the possibility of shock in any victim of an accident or when significant illness develops. Insure that an adequate airway is established (see further discussion under RESCUE BREATHING, page 19). Assess the cardiovascular status. Place your hand over the carotid artery (Figure 1) to obtain the pulse. In compensatory shock the patient will have a weak, rapid pulse. In adults the rate will be over 140, in children 180 beats per minute. If there is doubt about a pulse being present, listen to the bare chest. If cardiac standstill is present, begin one- person or two-person CPR (see page 20). Elevate the legs to 45° to obtain a better return of venous blood to the heart and head. However, if there has been a severe head injury, keep the person flat. If they have trouble breathing, elevate the chest and head to a comfortable position. Protect the patient from the environment with insulation under and shelter up above. Strive to make them comfortable. Watch your spoken and body language. Reassure without patronizing and let nothing that you say or act out cause them increased distress.

Attempt to treat the underlying cause of the shock. The primary or secondary survey and history may well elicit the cause of shock and appropriate treatment can be devised from the field expedient methods listed in this book.

Shock due to severe allergic reactions is called "anaphylactic shock" and is discussed on page 145.

DIFFICULT RESPIRATIONS

It has been stated that you can live three minutes without air, three days without water, three weeks without food, and three months without love. Some feel that these categories might stretch their time limits to four, others would feel shorter periods might be lethal. Without any question, adequate respirations are the most significant demand of the living creature. When respiratory difficulties start, it's urgent to find the reason and alleviate it. When they stop, reestablishing the airflow is critical.

DECISION/CARE TABLE

If no breathing is present - from whatever cause -
see RESCUE BREATHING, page 19

If no heart beat is present - from whatever cause -
see CARDIAC COMPRESSION, page 20

If associated with high altitude (above 6,500 feet) -
see HIGH ALTITUDE ILLNESS, page 194

If associated with cold conditions -
see HYPOTHERMIA, page 182

If body temperature is over 100° F with cough -
see PNEUMONIA/BRONCHITIS, page 61

If severe pain, sudden onset, after trauma -
see FRACTURED RIBS, page 143

If severe pain, sudden onset, no trauma -
see PNEUMOTHORAX, page 144
see PULMONARY EMBOLUS, page 62
see CARDIAC EVALUATION AND CARE, page 24

If associated with hysterical reaction -
see HYPERVENTILATION SYNDROME, page 23

If associated with choking -
see FOREIGN-BODY AIRWAY OBSTRUCTION, page 18

If associated with dull ache in middle of chest -
see CARDIAC EVALUATION AND CARE, page 24

FOREIGN BODY AIRWAY OBSTRUCTION

If a conscious adult seems to be having distress breathing, ask "Are you choking?" If they apparently are, perform a subdiaphragmatic abdominal thrust, also called an "abdominal thrust" or "Heimlich Maneuver," to relieve foreign-body airway obstruction, or choking. If the victim is standing or sitting, the rescuer stands behind and wraps his arms around the patient, proceeding as follows: Make a fist with one hand. Place the thumb side of the fist against the victim's abdomen, in the midline slightly above the navel and well below the breast bone (xiphoid process of the sternum). Grasp the fist with the other hand. Press the fist into the victim's abdomen with a quick upward thrust. Each new thrust should be a separate and distinct movement. It may be necessary to repeat the thrust multiple times to clear the airway. If the person is obese or pregnant, use chest thrusts in the same manner as just described, but with the hands around the lower chest.

If the victim becomes unconscious and is on the ground, the victim should be placed on their back, face up. In civilization activate the Emergency Medical Response system. Perform a tongue-jaw lift, followed by a finger sweep to remove the object. Open the airway and try to ventilate. If still obstructed, reposition the head and try to ventilate again. Give up to 5 abdominal thrusts, then repeat the tongue-jaw lift, finger sweep, and attempt at ventilation. Repeat these steps until effective.

To perform an abdominal thrust with the patient on the ground, the rescuer kneels astride the victim's thighs. The rescuer places the heel of one hand against the victim's abdomen, in the midline slightly above the navel and well below the breastbone, and the second hand directly on top of the first. The rescuer then presses into the abdomen with quick upward thrusts.

Were these maneuvers to fail with the debris located above the trachea, a tracheostomy would be life saving. Probably the best field expedient technique is the cricothyrotomy.

CRICOTHYROTOMY

If the patient is in imminent danger of dying from airway obstruction, the obstruction or damage being at a level of the larynx or above, a rapid field technique to provide an artificial airway that is very dangerous, but less so than the even more dangerous tracheostomy, is the cricothyrotomy. In essence, a hole is placed in the thin cricothyroid membrane and a hollow object shoved into the hole to keep an external airway open. This membrane stretches between the Adam's apple (thyroid cartilage) and the prominent ring just below the Adam's apple, called the cricoid cartilage.

With the patient lying on a flat surface, head extended, prepare the area with antiseptic if there is time. Povidone-iodine or alcohol prep pads would work well. Palpate for the cricothyroid membrane's location between the Adam's apple and cricoid cartilage. Make a vertical stab incision through the outer skin and the membrane. This opening will have to be kept from collapsing with the use of a hollow tube (such as a ball point pen casing, if nothing better is available.) Emergency department physicians have available to them a special cannula that they use in place of ball point pens. Any large bore needle may be used (12 or 14 gauge—the lower the number, the larger the needle bore.) After placement, the needle would have to be carefully taped into position to prevent dislodgment. Two needles can be placed side by side to provide better ventilation, especially if oxygen is not available to enrich the mixture the patient is breathing.

There are many complications that can result from this procedure - the esophagus can be punctured, the cricoid cartilage and first tracheal ring may be cut, the recurrent laryngeal nerve may be cut causing damage to the voice, and even the top of the lung can be punctured. (It is amazing how high in the neck the top portions of the lungs are located.)

If the patient recovers well enough not to require the cricothyrotomy any longer, just remove the needle or cannula and the wound will seal itself in short order. Even butterfly closures should prove adequate to approximate the wound.

ADULT ONE-RESCUER CPR

New techniques for CPR were published in 1992. Establish unresponsiveness, first by talking to the victim asking a question such as "Are you OK, are you OK?" If there is no response to your verbal contact, make gentle physical contact by touching the victim's shoulder and repeating your question. In civilization activate the EMS system prior to attempting CPR. In the wilderness immediately proceed with the following steps.

Open the airway using the head-tilt, chin-lift or jaw-thrust technique (see Figure 2). Place one hand on the victim's forehead and apply firm, backwards pressure with the palm to tilt the head back. Also place the fingers of the other hand under the bony part of the lower jaw near the chin and lift to bring the chin forward and the teeth almost shut, thus supporting the jaw and helping to tilt the head back, as indicated in Figure 2. In case of suspected neck injury, use the chin-lift without the head-tilt technique. The nose is pinched shut by using the thumb and index finger of the hand on the forehead.

The chin-lift method will place tension on the tongue and throat structures to insure that the air passage will open. This opening of the air passage may be all that is required to allow the victim to start breathing again. Reassess breathing again by looking for the chest raising or falling, listening for air escaping during expiration, and feeling the movement of air.

FIGURE 2.
The head-tilt, chin-lift method of opening the airway in an unconscious person.

If breathing is absent, give 2 slow breaths (1- to 2 seconds per breath), watching the chest rise. Then allow for exhalation between breaths. The breathing rate should be once every 5 to 6 seconds, about 12 breaths per minute. Using slow, full breaths reduces the amount of air that tends to enter the stomach which causes gastric distention. Watch the victim's chest rise and allow for exhalation between breaths.

Check the carotid pulse. This is found by placing your hand on the voice box (larynx). Slip the tips of your fingers into the groove beside the voice box and feel for the pulse. (see Figure 1). If breathing is absent but pulse is present, provide rescue breathing at the rate of about 12 breaths per minute. If there is no pulse, give cycles of 15 chest compressions (at a rate of 80 to 100 compressions per minute), followed by 2 slow breaths.

Chest compressions are performed by the rescuer kneeling at the victim's side, near his chest, locating the notch at the lowest portion of his breast bone (sternum). Place the heel of one hand on the sternum 1- to 2 inches above this notch, Place the other hand on top of the one that is in position on the sternum. Be sure to keep your fingers off the ribs. The easiest way to prevent this is to interlock your fingers, thus keeping them confined to the sternum. With your shoulders directly over the victim's sternum, compress downward keeping your arms straight. Depress the sternum 1- to 2 inches for an average adult victim. Relax the pressure completely, keeping your hands in contact with the sternum at all times, but allowing the sternum to return to its normal position between compressions. Both compression and relaxation should be of equal duration.

Perform 15 external chest compressions at a rate of 80 to 100 per minute. Open the airway and deliver 2 rescue breaths. Locate the proper

FIGURE 3.

Position of hands.   *Position of rescuer.*

hand position and begin 15 more compressions at a rate of 80 to 100 per minute, then 2 slow breaths. Perform 4 complete cycles of 15 compressions followed by 2 slow breaths.

After 4 cycles of 15:2 compressions and ventilations (about 1 minute), reevaluate the patient. Check for the return of the carotid pulse (5 seconds). If it is absent, resume CPR with 15 compressions followed by 2 slow breaths, as indicated above. If it is present, continue to the next step.

Check breathing (3 to 5 seconds). If present, monitor breathing and pulse closely. If absent, perform rescue breathing at 12 times per minute and monitor pulse closely.

If CPR is continued, stop and check for return of pulse and spontaneous breathing after each 4 cycles. Do not interrupt CPR for more than 5 seconds except in special circumstances.

Once CPR is started it should be maintained until professional assistance can take over the responsibility, or until a physician declares the patient dead. In the wilderness, if CPR has been continued for 30 minutes without regaining cardiac function and the eyes are fixed and nonreactive to light, the patient can be presumed dead. The exceptions would be hypothermia (see page 182) and lightning injuries (page 191). In these circumstances CPR should be continued until the rescuers are exhausted if professional help does not intervene.

Some authorities in wilderness rescue have felt that the survival rate is so low without defibrillation within 4 minutes by paramedics, that CPR should not be started in the bush when cardiac standstill is due to a heart attack. It certainly should not be started or maintained under these conditions when its performance might endanger the lives of members of the rescue party. Regardless, learning CPR is an important skill that every person should master. THE ONLY WAY TO LEARN THIS TECHNIQUE IS TO TAKE A CPR COURSE—IT CANNOT BE PROPERLY SELF-TAUGHT.

ADULT TWO-RESCUER CPR

The two-rescuer technique differs in that rescuer 1 will take a position by the head and rescuer 2 assumes the position as described under one-rescuer CPR. While breathing and compression rates are the same, the ratios are different.

After establishing unresponsiveness (and activating the EMS system if in civilization), rescuer 1 opens the airway (head-tilt, chin-lift or jaw-thrust) and checks for breathing (look, feel, listen). Rescuer 1 then gives 2 slow breaths (1½ to 2 seconds per breath), watches the chest rise, and allows for exhalation between breaths. After the 2 breaths, rescuer 1 checks the carotid pulse.

If there is no pulse, rescuer 2 gives cycles of 5 chest compressions (rate of 80 to 100 compressions per minute), followed by 1 slow breath by rescuer 1. After 1 minute of rescue support, rescuer 1 again checks the pulse. If there is no pulse, this 5:1 compression breathing cycle is continued, with periodic reassessment.

Two person CPR is not generally taught to the public in basic courses to avoid confusion with the ratios and rates of the compressions and respirations of one person CPR. However, in the wilderness where prolonged CPR might be necessary, being familiar with this technique can help alleviate the tremendous fatigue which CPR induces in rescuers.

RAPID BREATHING

HYPERVENTILATION SYNDROME, TACHYPNEA: Rapid breathing (hyperventilation or tachypnea) can represent either a serious medical condition or can be the result of a harmless panic attack. This symptom in a diabetic is very dangerous, but can be prevented by proper diabetic management. High altitude stress can result in hyperventilation (see page 194). See the table on page 18 for additional diagnosis of a rapid or difficult breathing disorder.

A feeling of panic which results in very rapid shallow breathing causes the victim to lose excessive amounts of carbon dioxide from the bloodstream. The resulting change in the acid-base balance of the blood (respiratory alkalosis) will cause a numb feeling around the mouth, in the extremities, and if the breathing pattern persists, it can even lead to violent spasms of the hands and feet. This is a form of hysteria which can appear in teenagers and healthy young adults. It would be helpful for victims to re-breathe their air from a stuff sack to increase the carbon dioxide level in their bloodstream. They need to be reassured and told to slow down the breathing. It is fine for them to draw long, deep breaths as it is the rapid breathing that causes the loss of so much carbon dioxide.

If necessary, from the Non-Rx Oral Medication Module give Percogesic 2 tablets or from the Rx Oral/Topical Medication Module give Atarax 25mg, 2 tablets. Or the Rx Injectable Module medication Vistaril 50 mg IM is helpful in treating hyperventilation. These drugs are being used in this instance as anti-anxiety drugs.

CARDIAC EVALUATION AND CARE

HEART ATTACK - MYOCARDIAL INFARCTION: The symptoms of chest heaviness or pain with exertion; pain or ache radiating into the neck or into the arms; sweating, clammy, pale appearance; and/or shortness of breath are fairly classic for a person having an inadequate oxygen supply to the heart. The pain is called "angina" and results from the heart muscle starving for oxygen. If the blockage is profound, heart muscle will die. This is called a "myocardial infarction" and it means heart attack and damaged muscle. The cause of death is frequently a profound irregular heart beat caused by electrical irritation in the damaged muscle. Another cause of death is loss of adequate power to pump blood from weakened heart muscle. A delayed cause of death can be from the sudden rupture of the weakened heart wall.

The only thing which can be done for this individual in the wilderness is rest. Rest causes the oxygen requirement of the heart to be at a minimum. Position the victim for optimum comfort, generally with his head elevated about 45 degrees. In some cases, even with an electrocardiogram, it is impossible for a trained physician to determine whether or not an individual is having a cardiac problem. When in doubt - rest the patient and try to evacuate without having him do any of the work. Treat as a total invalid.

Check to see if the victim is carrying any prescription heart medications and note usage instructions on the bottle. Give sublingual nitroglycerin if anyone in the party is carrying it. One tablet, followed by two more at 5 minute intervals would be appropriate. You may give the victim medication adequate to relieve pain (see page 30). From the Rx oral module give Atarax (hydroxyzine) 25 mg orally, or from the Rx injection module Vistaril (hydroxyzine) 25 mg IM, if needed to treat nausea or to help sedate the victim. You may repeat the pain medication and the nausea/sedation medication every 4 hours as needed.

Observe respirations and pulse rate. You will note the comment in the section under Adult-One Rescuer CPR that providing CPR to a heart attack victim who cannot be defibrillated within 4 minutes is a lost cause. The only significant reason for starting CPR, if the person becomes pulseless, is to placate the onlookers. Due to the virtual zero salvage rate, you are treating yourself and the others watching who, after perhaps one-half hour, will consider that everything had been done that was possible. This attempt may be a very important part of the emotional support required by individual group members as they reflect back upon the event.

RAPID HEART RATE

TACHYCARDIA: A rapid heart rate after trauma or other stress may signify impending shock. The underlying cause should be treated. This may require fluid replacement or pain medication. Body temperature elevations cause an increase in heart rate of 10 beats per minute for each degree above normal. At elevations above 8,000 feet (2,500 meters), a pulse rate of 120 or greater per minute after a 20 minute rest is an early sign of pulmonary edema. A sudden onset of rapid heart rate with sharp chest pain can indicate a pulmonary embolism or pneumothorax.

A very rapid rate of 140 to 220 beats per minute may be encountered suddenly and without warning in very healthy individuals. This PAT (paroxysmal atrial tachycardia) has as its first symptom, frequently, a feeling of profound weakness. The victim generally stops what she is doing and feels better sitting down. These attacks are self-limited, but they can be aborted by one of several maneuvers which stimulate the vagus nerve which in turn slows down the pulse rate. These maneuvers include: holding one's breath and bearing down very hard; closing one's eyes and pressing firmly on the eyeballs; inducing vomiting with a finger down the throat; or feeling for the carotid pulse in the neck and gently pressing on the enlarged portion of this vessel, one side at a time. Another effective maneuver is to take a deep breath and plunge one's face into ice water. Frequently, however, the victim must just wait for the attack to pass. This arrhythmia will sometimes come on after a spate of activity. No medication is generally required.

SLOW HEART RATE

BRADYCARDIA: A slow heart rate is important in two instances: when associated with passing out and when accompanied by high fever. Generally fainting or shock is associated with a rapid pulse rate (see compensatory shock, page 17) in an attempt by the body to maintain blood pressure. A safety mechanism which the body employs to prevent blood pressure from going too high is a sensor system in each carotid artery called the carotid body. If this sensor is stimulated by the pressure going through the artery raising too high, a reflex mechanism which opens blood vessels and lowers the heart rate is brought into play via the vagus nerve. The vagus nerve can be fooled into inappropriately initiating this reflex mechanism at times. A person watching an accident scene, or even thinking about such an episode, can stimulate the vagus nerve through its connection with the frontal lobe. The resulting slow pulse and relaxed arteries can result in the person passing out.

As mentioned on page 25, the pulse usually increases as the body temperature rises. It also falls as the core temperature lowers into a hypothermic state (see page 182). Several diseases are notable in that the pulse rate is lower than would be expected for the elevated body temperature caused by the disease. To illustrate this point, a typical example of such a disease is typhoid fever.

TYPHOID FEVER

Besides the slow pulse rate, this disease is characterized by headache, chills, loss of appetite, back ache, constipation, nosebleed, and tenderness of the abdomen to palpation. The temperature rises daily for 7 to 10 days. The fever is maintained at a high level for 7 to 19 more days, then drops over the next 10 days. With typhoid fever, a pulse rate of only 84 may occur with a temperature of 104 degrees Fahrenheit. Between the 7th and 10th day of illness, rose-colored splotches, which blanche when pressure is applied, appear in 10% of patients. The drug of choice for this illness is Rocephin, given 30 mg/kg of body weight/day IM in two divided doses per day for two weeks. An oral drug that can be used is Floxin 400 mg given twice daily. Diarrhea may become important in the latter stages of this illness. Replacement of fluids is especially important during the phases of high fever or diarrhea (see page 70). Patients with relapses should be given another 5-day course of the antibiotic. Immunization prior to departure to endemic areas is useful in curtailing the severity of this infection (see page 223).

BODY SYSTEM SYMPTOMS AND MANAGEMENT

SYMPTOM MANAGEMENT

Symptoms are indicators of problems. Such things as fever, pain, and itch can sometimes aid you in determining exactly what is wrong with the patient. You will note that various decision tables in this book will use one or more symptoms to help identify a diagnosis and treatment course.

It is also useful to know how to minimize some of these symptoms. Why itch when you can treat it? The diagnosis may vary from poison plant dermatitis and insect bite to liver disease, but regardless of the cause, what can you do to alleviate it?

The best method of alleviating symptoms is to successfully treat the underlying problem. Sometimes definitive treatment cannot be accomplished. At other times, the symptom remains after the injury is past and the symptom becomes the greatest part of the problem.

The following sections provide a guide to general symptom care.

Breathing difficulties, see page 17

Cough, see page 61

Diarrhea, see page 67

Fever/Chills, see page 28

Heart rate, too fast, see page 25

Hiccups, see page 33

Itch, see page 32

Lethargy, see page 29

Nausea/vomiting, see page 66

Pain, see page 30

For a discussion of symptoms localized to a particular body part, refer to the anatomical location listings later in the section or the body location and symptom cross referenced in the Clinical Reference Index starting on page 231. Evaluation and management of symptoms relating to injuries and environmental exposure can also be found through the Clinical Reference Index.

FEVER, CHILLS

The average oral temperature of a resting individual is 98.6° 99.6° F (37° C), while in active individuals 101° F (38° C). Rectal temperatures are 0.5 to 1° F higher. A temperature rise in a human will result in the heart rate increasing 10 beats per minute faster than the patient's normal resting temperature. This is a useful field method of judging temperature, if each individual knows what his resting pulse is. Some diseases cause a peculiar drop in heart rate even in the face of an obviously high temperature. The most notable of these is typhoid fever, page 26 and yellow fever, page 180.

Although injury and exposure can cause elevated body temperature, fever is usually the result of infection. The cause of the fever should be sought and treated. If pain or infection is located in the ear, throat, etc., refer to the appropriate anatomical area listed in the Clinical Reference Index at the end of the book (starting on page 231).

If other symptoms beside fever are present (diarrhea, cough, etc.), see the cross references listing these symptoms in the Clinical Reference Index in order to provide treatment to alleviate the suffering of these conditions. This may diagnose the underlying disease which would have a specific treatment indicated in the text.

The wilderness approach to therapy may be quite different from that used in clinical medicine. In the wilderness when in doubt about whether or not the fever is due to viral, bacterial, or other infectious causes, treat with antibiotic from your Rx medical modules. Initially, give the patient Cefzil™ 250 mg, 1 tablet every 12 hours and continue until the fever has broken and then reduce the dosage to 1 tablet daily for an additional 4 days. This will conserve medication while providing adequate antibiotic coverage to a suspected bacterial infection. If it is possible that the patient has a strep throat (see page 54), continue coverage for a total of 10 days. If you are not carrying the Rx kit, then treat the symptoms using the medications described in your non-Rx kits. In either case, rest is important until the patient is again free of fever and has a sense of well being.

Chills are a state of shivering with a sense of coldness—not related to hypothermia as discussed on page 182. Chills are usually followed by fever. They frequently indicate the onset of a bacterial infection which should be treated with an antibiotic as described above.

People tolerate fevers quite well and it is possible that elevated temperatures enhance the immune response to infections. Persons with a history of febrile seizures and persons with a history of heart problems should certainly be treated to lower an elevated temperature. Generally it is best to use Tylenol™ (acetaminophen), but usually ibuprofen and aspirin are safe. Aspirin should be avoided in children with chicken pox or other viral illness due to an increase in Reye's syndrome with its use (a disease of progressive liver failure and brain deterioration). The Non-Rx Oral Medication Module contains two products useful in treating fever, ibuprofen and Percogesic. As these are over the counter products, the dosage will be listed on the product containers.

LETHARGY

Lethargy, or prolonged tiredness or malaise, is a non-localizing symptom such as fever or muscle ache (myalgia). Pain, however, is a localizing symptom that points to the organ system which may be the cause of such things as lethargy, fever, or a generally ill feeling. Frequently after a brief period of a few days of lethargy - or at times even hours - localizing symptoms develop and the cause of the lethargy can be determined to be an infection of the throat, ear, etc.

Sometimes a chronic condition is the source of the lethargy, such as anemia, leukemia, low thyroid function, depression, occult or low grade infection, mental depression, or even physical exhaustion. The latter we would expect to be obvious from the history of the preceding level of activity and strength should return within a few days.

Anemia can present due to chronic blood loss from ulcers, menstrual problems, lack of adequate formation due to low iron, leukemia and other cancers in the bone marrow, etc. A chronic anemia can be identified by looking at the color of the skin inside the lower eye lids. Pull the lower lid down and look at it. Compare to another person. Normally this thin skin is very orange colored, even if the cheeks are pale. If the color is a blanched, white - then anemia is very likely. Another good indication of anemia is an increase in the pulse rate of more than 30 beats per minute in the standing position compared to the prone (or laying down) position.

Malaise or lethargy can be a presenting complaint of acute mountain sickness, but this would be unusual below 6,000 feet. If other symptoms are present such as nausea, one must think of hepatitis (see page 168), or if preceded by a severe sore throat then infectious mononucleosis (see page 54). Lethargy is one of the most common presenting complaints which I see in my office. The full length of possible diagnosis is lengthy and requires careful evaluation and, frequently, laboratory tests. If the problem is not depression, then regardless of the cause, the person needs rest, proper nutrition, and adequate shelter.

PAIN

Adequate pain management can be a mixture of proper medication and attitude—the attitude of both the victim and the medic being important. A calm, professional approach to problems will lessen anxiety, panic, and pain. Pain is an important symptom that tells you something is wrong. It generally "localizes" or points to the exact cause of the trouble, so that pain in various parts of the body will be your clue that a problem exists and that specific treatment may be required to eliminate it. Refer to the Clinical Reference Index (page 231) for areas of the body (such as ear, abdomen, etc.) where pain exists to read further about diagnosis and for further specific treatments of the causes of pain.

An application of cold water or ice can frequently relieve pain. This is very important in burns, orthopedic injuries, and skin irritations. Cold can sometimes relieve muscle spasm. Gentle massage and local hot compresses are also effective treatments for muscle spasm.

The alleviation of pain with medication calls for a step-wise increase in medication strength until relief is obtained. Throughout this book you will be referred to this section for adequate pain management. Use discretion in providing adequate medication to do the job, without overdosing the patient. Remember that a pill takes about 20 minutes to begin working and is at maximum therapeutic strength in about one hour. If possible, wait an hour to see how effective the medication has been. But use common sense. If the injury is severe, give a respectable initial dose.

For mild pain, from the Non-Rx Oral Medication Module provide the victim with Percogesic, 1 or 2 tablets every 4 hours. Percogesic is probably the best pain medication that can be obtained without a prescription, providing both pain and muscle relaxant actions. It is fully described on page 205. It is particularly good for orthopedic injuries or whenever muscle sprains and contusions are encountered. It is also ideal for menstrual cramps, tension headache, and it is relatively safe to use in head injuries. It can also be used for the muscle aches and fever from viral and bacterial infections.

Another pain medication suggested in the Non-Rx Oral Medication Module is ibuprofen. Its anti-inflammatory abilities make it ideal for treatment of tendinitis, bursitis, or arthritic pain. Brand names generally available are Nuprin, Medipren, and Advil. An alternate selection for this product would be either a buffered aspirin or enteric coated aspirin product.

For SEVERE PAIN you may have to rely on the Rx Oral/Topical Medication Module component Lorcet 10/650, taking 1 tablet every 4 to 6 hours. One of these tablets is generally enough to eliminate a bad toothache in a large adult. The total 24 hour dose should not exceed 6 tablets. They can be augmented by also giving the victim 1 or 2 Atarax 25 mg tablets every 4 to 6 hours. This medication helps eliminate the nausea associated with high hydrocodone dosages and from my experience it also potentiates the pain medication so that it works more effectively.

The Rx Oral/Topical Medication Module also contains nasal inhaled Stadol® (butorphanol tartrate). This very powerful pain medication is about 10 times stronger per milligram dose than morphine. It is taken as a spray up one nostril, followed by another spray in the other nostril in 5 to 20 minutes if necessary. This may be repeated every 3 to 4 hours. This medication is as powerful as any injectable product available. See full discussion of this medication on page 212. Its rate of onset is fairly rapid. Within 5 minutes relief should start with maximum effect being obtained within 20 minutes. As there are no needles required to administer this drug, it should be easier to take on foreign trips than the injectable medications. You might consider keeping it with your toothpaste until across the border. At least I do.

If you are carrying the Rx Injection Module, severe pain can be treated with an injection of 10 mg of Nubain® (nalbuphine). This amounts to ½ ml of the strength listed in the kit. This can be potentiated with Vistaril® (hydroxyzine) 25 mg or 50 mg, also by injection. Vistaril and Nubain can be mixed in the same syringe. They both sting upon injection.

Local pain can be eliminated with cold compresses or ice as mentioned above. Applying dibucaine 1% ointment will help skin surface pain, such as from sunburn, abrasions, etc. Applying a cover of Spenco 2nd Skin® dressing (both products are recommended for the Non-Rx Topical Bandaging Module) provides cooling relief due to the evaporative action of the water from this safe to use gel pad. Deep cuts and painful puncture wounds can be injected with lidocaine 1% from the Rx Injectable Medical Module. This technique is described on page 95.

ITCH

As itch is a sensation that is transmitted by pain fibers, all pain medications can be used in alleviating itch sensations. Itch is also an indication of something being awry and possibly requiring specific treatment. The most common causes are local allergic reactions, such as poisonous plants (page 111), fungal infections (page 110), and insect bites or infestations (pages 154-157) or look under specific causes in the index). General principles of treatment include further avoidance of the offending substance (not so easy in the case of mosquitoes). Avoid applying heat to an itchy area, as this flares it worse. Avoid scratching or rubbing, this also increases the reaction. If weeping blisters have formed, apply wet soaks with a clean cloth or gauze. While plain water soaks will help, making a solution of boric acid, epsom salts, or even regular table salt will help dry the lesions and alleviate some of the itch. Make an approximately 10% solution weight to volume of water.

Cream-based preparations work well on moist lesions, while ointments are more effective on dry, scaly ones. The Non-Rx Topical/Bandaging Module contains 1% hydrocortisone cream which, while safe to use, is generally not very effective against severe allergic dermatitis. To potentiate it, one should apply it four times daily and then cover the area with an occlusive dressing, such as cellophane or a piece of polybag. The Rx Oral/Topical Medication Module contains Topicort® (desoximetasone) .25% cream, which is strong enough to adequately treat allergic dermatitis with light coats applied twice daily. Athlete's foot and skin rashes in the groin or in skinfolds are generally fungal and should not be treated with these creams. They may seem to provide temporary relief, but they can actually worsen fungal infections. For possible fungal infections, apply the clotrimazole cream 1% twice daily from the Non-Rx Topical/Bandaging Module.

Oral medications are frequently required to treat severe skin reactions and itch. The Non-Rx Oral Medication Module contains Benadryl® (diphenhydramine) 25 mg. Take 1 or 2 capsules every 6 hours. It is one of the most effective antihistamines made. The Rx Oral Medication Module contains Atarax® (hydroxyzine) 25 mg. Atarax is very effective in treating the symptom of itch and in its other anti-histamine actions. Take 1 or 2 tablets every 6 hours. These medications are safe to use on all sorts of itch problems. If one is suffering from an asthma attack they should not be used, however, as they tend to dry out the lung secretions and potentially make the illness worse.

Hives are the result of a severe allergic reaction. Commonly called welts, these raised red blotches develop rapidly and frequently have a red border around a clearer skin area in the center, sometimes referred to as an "annular" lesion. As these can and do appear over large surfaces of the skin, treatment with a cream is of little help. Use the Benadryl or Atarax as indicated above. Extensive urticaria or allergic dermatitis lesions frequently need to be treated with an oral steroid. The Rx Oral/Topical Medication Module has Decadron® (dexamethasone) 4 mg tablets, which should be taken 1 tablet twice daily after meals.

It should be noted that the Vistaril® recommended for the Rx Injectable Module is also hydroxyzine as is the oral Atarax. This same module also has an injectable form of the Decadron. For treatment of rash, the oral medications should suffice.

In case of a concurrent asthmatic condition or the development of shock, treat as indicated under "anaphylactic shock" on page 145. In case of suspected tick bite, an annular lesion may be a sign of Lyme disease (see page 169). If fever is present, one must consider that the rash and itch has resulted from an infection. A diagnosis may be impossible in the bush so that treatment with antibiotic is appropriate. Use Cefzil 250 mg twice daily from the Rx Oral/Topical Medication Module as a field expedient solution to the problem. Treat fever as described in that section on page 28.

HICCUPS

Hiccups can be started by a variety of causes and are generally self-limited. Persistent hiccups can be a medically important symptom requiring professional evaluation and help in control. Several approaches to their control in camp may be tried. Have the victim hold his breath for as long as possible or re-breathe air from a stuff sack. These maneuvers raise the carbon dioxide level and help stop the hiccup reflex mechanism. Drinking 5 to 6 ounces of ice water fast sometimes works; one may also close his eyes and press firmly on the eyeballs to stimulate the vagal blockage of the hiccup. The other vagus nerve stimulation maneuvers indicated under PAT, page 25, can be tried.

If these maneuvers do not work, from the Non-Rx Oral Medication Module give Percogesic 2 tablets or from the Rx Oral/Topical Medication Module you may give Atarax 25 mg, 2 tablets. The Rx Injectable Module medication Vistaril 50 mg IM is also effective for this condition. These doses may be repeated every 4 hours. Let the patient rest and try to avoid bothering him until bedtime. If still symptomatic at that point, have him re-breathe the air from inside his sleeping bag, to raise the carbon dioxide level in his blood stream and, if nothing else, to muffle the sounds.

EYE PROBLEMS

Pain and irritation of the eye can be devastating. Causes which might be encountered in a remote area trip are listed in the table below.

TABLE 1					
SYMPTOMS AND SIGNS OF EYE PATHOLOGY					
	Vision Loss	**Pain**	**Red**	**Drainage**	**Tissue Swelling**
Trauma *(Page 44)*	x	xx	xx	x	x
Foreign Body *(Page 35)*		xx	xx	xx	
Infection *(Page 41)*					
bacteria		x	xx	xx	x
viral		x	xx	x	x
sty		x	xx		xx
Allergy *(Page 43)*			xx	x	
Corneal Ulcers *(Page 38)*	x	xx			
Snow Blindness *(Page 40)*	x	xx	xx	x	
Strain		x			
Glaucoma *(Page 45)*	x	xx			
Spontaneous *(Page 44)*					
Subconjunctival			xx		
Hemorrhage					

xx = A frequent or intense symptom
x = Common, less intense symptom
Blank = Less likely to produce this symptom

EYE PATCH AND BANDAGING TECHNIQUES

In case of evidence of infection, do not use an eye patch or splint, but have the patient wear dark glasses, a wide brimmed hat, or take other measures to decrease light exposure. Wash the eye with clean water by dabbing with a wet, clean cloth, every two hours to remove pus and excess secretions. Apply antibiotics as indicated under eye infections.

Eye patch techniques must allow for gentle closure of the eyelid and retard blinking activity. Sometimes both eyes must be patched for this to succeed, but this obviously is a hardship for the patient. Simple strips of tape holding the eyelids shut may suffice. In case of trauma, an annular ring of cloth may be constructed to pad the eye without pressure over the eyeball. A simple eye patch with oversize gauze or cloth may work fine, as the bone of the orbital rim around the eye acts to protect the eyeball which is recessed.

Serious injury requires patching both eyes, as movement in the injured eye will decrease if movement in the unaffected eye is also controlled. It generally helps to have the victim kept in a 30° head elevated position and at rest after eye injury. A severe blow to one eye may cause temporary blindness in both eyes which can resolve in hours to days. Obviously, a person with loss of vision should be treated by a physician if possible. Eye dressings must be removed, or at least changed, in 24 hours.

If the victim has suffered a corneal abrasion, or after removing foreign bodies, the best splint is the tension patch. Start by placing two gauze pads over the shut eye, requesting the patient to keep his eyes closed until the bandaging is completed. The patient may help hold the gauze in place. Three pieces of one inch wide tape are ideal, long enough to extend from the center of the forehead to just below the cheek bone. Fasten the first piece of tape to the center of the forehead, extending the tape diagonally downward across the eye patch. The second and third strips are applied parallel to the first strip, one above and the other below. This dressing will result in firm splinting of the bandaged eye.

FOREIGN BODY, EYE

The most common eye problems in the wilderness will be foreign body, abrasion, snow blindness and infection (conjunctivitis). Therapy for these problems is virtually the same, except that it is very important to remove any foreign body that may be present.

The initial step in examining the painful eye is to remove the pain. One of the lessons drilled into medical students is to never, never write a prescription for eye anesthesia agents (such as the Tetracaine .5% ophthalmic (eye) drops which I recommend for the Rx Oral/Topical Medication Module). The reason is the patient may use it, obtain relief, and then not have the eye carefully examined for a foreign body. Eventually, this foreign body may cause an ulcer to form in the cornea doing profound damage. When using the Tetracaine .5% ophthalmic drops, remember that it is very important to find and remove any foreign body. Use one or two drops and have the patient close his eye and let him rest with it shut, thus giving time for the medication to melt and anesthetize the eye. This medication burns when initially placed in the eye. This will increase the level of pain for a brief period until the medication takes effect. After the patient has calmed down, have him open the eye and look straight ahead. Very carefully shine a pen light at the cornea from one side to see if a minute speck becomes visible. By moving the light back and forth, one might see movement of a shadow on the iris of the eye and thus confirm the presence of a foreign body.

In making the foreign body examination, also be sure to check under the eyelids. Evert the upper lid over a Q-tip stick, thus examining not only the eyeball, but also the undersurface of the eyelid. This surface may be gently brushed with the cotton applicator to eliminate minute particles. Always use a fresh Q-tip when touching the eye or eyelid each additional time. Some foreign bodies can be removed easily. Have the patient place his face under water and blink. Water turbulence from underwater blinking or turbulence from directing running water from a fast moving stream or by pouring from a cup may wash the problem away.

When a foreign body has been identified which is imbedded in the cornea, take a sterile, or at least a clean, Q-tip and approach the foreign body from the side. Gently prod it with the Q-tip handle until it is loosened. The surface of the eye will indent under the pressure of this scraping action. Indeed the surface of the cornea will be scratched in the maneuver, but it will quickly heal. Once the foreign body has been dislodged, if it does not stick to the wooden or plastic handle, but slides loose along the corneal surface, use the cotton portion to touch it for removal.

A stoic individual, particularly one accustomed to contact lenses, might be able to undergo a non-complicated foreign body removal without the use of Tetracaine .5% ophthalmic drops, but using anesthesia makes the patient more comfortable and cuts down on interference from the blink reflex.

Foreign bodies stuck in the cornea can be very stubborn and resist removal. At times it is necessary to pick them loose with the sharp point of a #11 scalpel blade or the tip of a needle (I frequently use an 18 gauge needle). Anesthesia with Tetracaine 0.5% ophthalmic drops will be a necessity for this procedure. Scraping with these instruments will cause a more significant scrape to the corneal surface, but under these circumstances it may have to be accepted. I would leave stubborn foreign bodies for removal by a physician in all but the most desperate circumstances. If you have a difficult time removing an obvious foreign body from the surface of the cornea, a wait of two to three days may allow the cornea to ulcerate slightly so that removal with the Q-tip stick may be much easier. Deeply lodged foreign bodies will have to be left for surgical removal.

A painless foreign body may not be a foreign body. It could be a rust ring left behind after a bit of ferrous, or iron containing, material has fallen out of the eye after having been lodged for a short time. If what you see is painless, ignore it in the wilderness setting.

The history of striking objects may indicate a deeper penetration than one would expect from blowing debris. A puncture wound of the eyelid mandates careful examination of the cornea surface for evidence of a penetrating foreign body. These injuries must be seen by a physician for surgical care. Evacuation is necessary. If this is impossible, the eye must be patched, examined for infection twice daily, and treated with antibiotic both by mouth and with ointment.

After removal of a foreign body, or even after scraping the eye while attempting to remove one, instill some antibiotic. The prescription kit should contain Tobrax ophthalmic ointment in a ⅛ oz tube. This is instilled by pulling down on the lower lid and laying a ribbon along the everted margin. Have the patient close the eye to allow the medication to melt. In the same manner apply a small amount of the Tetracaine .5% ophthalmic drops to provide pain relief. Tetracaine .5% ophthalmic drops should not be used more than 4 times a day and for no longer than two days. Continued use may hinder the natural healing process and may disguise a significant injury or mask the presence of an additional foreign body. The prescription analgesic Lorcet 10/650 1 tablet every 4 to 6 hours, may be given for pain.

There are no nonprescription eye antibiotics. Brand name Neosporin and Polysporin ointments in 15 gram tubes are non-prescription antibiotics that can be used in the eye. However, the manufacturer cannot recommend the use of these over the counter products for this purpose. Percogesic or ibuprofen 200 mg, 2 tablets every 4 to 6 hours may be provided for pain.

CONTACT LENSES

The increased popularity of contact lens wear means that several problems associated with their use have also increased. The lenses are of two basic types. The hard, or rigid, lens which generally is smaller and does not extend beyond the iris, and the soft lens which does extend beyond the iris onto the white of the eye. Soft lenses have been designed for extended wear. Hard lens use requires frequent removal, as the delicate cornea of the eye obtains oxygen from the environment and nutrient from eye secretions. These lenses interfere with this process and therefore are detrimental to the cornea. Examine the eyes of all unconscious persons for the existence of hard lenses and remove them if found. It is probably best to remove soft lenses also as some are not designed for extended use and may also damage the eye.

Leaving most hard contact lenses in the eyes longer than 12 hours can result in corneal ulceration. While not serious, this can be a very painful experience. At times even an iritis may result. This condition almost always resolves on its own within one day. The history is the major clue that the diagnosis is correct. If the condition failed to clear within 24 hours, other problems should be looked into such as corneal laceration, foreign body, or eye infection. After removal of the contact lens, place cool cloths on the eyes or ice packs to the eyes. This patient should be evaluated by a physician to confirm the diagnosis. Provide protection from sunlight. Patching both eyes while at rest will be of help. Give aspirin or other pain medication if available. The patient may have pain from the migration of the lens into one of the recesses of the conjunctiva, or possibly only have noted a loss of refractive correction. At times the complaint is a sudden "I have lost my contact lens!" Never forget to look in the eye as the possible hiding spot for the lens. Examine the eye as described in the section on foreign bodies in the eye. When dealing with a hard lens, use topical anesthesia as described if necessary and available. If the lens is loose, slide it over the pupil and allow the patient to remove it as they usually do. If the lens is adherent, rinse with eye irrigation solution or clean water and try again. If a corneal abrasion exists, patch as indicated above after the lens is removed.

The soft lens may generally be squeezed between the fingers and literally "popped" off. A special rubber pincer is sold that can aid in this maneuver. Hard lenses may also be removed with a special rubber suction cup device.

If the patient is unconscious, the hard lens will have to be removed. Lacking the suction cup device there are two different maneuvers which may be employed. One is the vertical technique. In this method, move the lens to the center of the eye over the pupil. Then press down on the lower lid, over the lower edge of the contact lens. Next squeeze the eyelids together, thus popping the lens out between them as indicated in Figure 4. In the lateral technique, the lens is slid to the outside corner of the eye. By tugging on the facial skin near the eye in a downward and outward direction, the lens can pop over the skin edge and be easily removed. See Figure 5.

The unconscious patient should have antibiotic salve placed in her eye and the lids taped or patched shut to prevent drying. These patches should be removed when needed for neurological checks, and certainly upon regaining consciousness.

If removal of the lens must be prolonged, safe storage will have to be provided. With regard to hard lenses, the ideal would be marked containers that pad the lens in such a way that they would not rattle around or otherwise become scratched. Small vials, labelled R and L, filled with a fluff of clean material, tapped together and placed in a safe location, would be ideal. Soft contact lenses must be protected from dehydration. It is always proper to store them in normal saline. This solution can be prepared by adding 1½ oz table salt to 1 pint of water. Of course, if the patient has a special solution for her lenses in her possession, use it.

FIGURE 4. *Contact lens removal—vertical technique.*

FIGURE 5. *Contact lens removal—horizontal technique.*

EYE ABRASION

Abrasions may be caused by a glancing blow from a wood chip, a swinging branch, even from blowing dirt, embers, ice or snow. The involved eye should be anesthetized with Rx Tetracaine .5% ophthalmic drops and protected with the Rx Tobrax ophthalmic ointment. Make sure that a foreign body has not been overlooked.

In cold wind be sure to protect your eyes from the effects of both blowing particles of ice and the wind itself. Grey Owl, in his interesting book, *Tales from an Empty Cabin*, tells how he was walking on one of his long trips through the backwoods along a windswept frozen lake when suddenly he lost sight of the tree line. He felt that he must be in a white-out, so he turned perpendicular to the wind and hiked toward the shore. Suddenly he bumped into a tree and realized that he was blind! He saved himself only by digging a snow cave and staying put for three days. He wondered how many good woodsmen were lost on their trap lines by such a similar incident, apparently a temporary opacification of the cornea from the cold wind or ice crystal abrasions.

SNOW BLINDNESS

This severely painful condition is primarily caused by ultraviolet B rays of the sun which are considerably reflected by snow (85%), water (10-100%), and sand (17%). Thin cloud layers allow the transmission of this wavelength, while filtering out infrared (heat) rays of the sun. Thus, it is possible on a rather cool, overcast day with bright snow conditions to become sunburned or snow blind.

Properly approved (ANSI) sunglasses will block 99.8% of the ultraviolet B wavelength. Suitable glasses should be tagged as meeting these standards.[5] Non-prescription glasses must be proper fitting and ideally provide side protection. A suitable retention strap must be worn, as I finally learned while rafting on the Green River in Colorado. And for those of us who must learn these things more than once, a second pair of glasses—particularly if prescription lenses are worn—is essential. Lacking sunglasses, any field expedient method of eliminating glare, such as slit glasses made from wood or any material at hand, to include the ubiquitous bandanna, will help. An important aspect of snow blindness is the delayed onset of symptoms. The pain and loss of vision may not be evident until after damaging exposure has been sustained.

Snow blindness is a self-limiting affliction. However, not only is the actually loss of vision a problem, but so is the terrible pain, usually described as feeling like red hot pokers were massaging the eye sockets. Lacking any first aid supplies the treatment would be a gentle eye patch and the application of cold packs as needed for pain relief. Generally both eyes are equally affected with a virtual total loss of vision. If there is partial sight and the party is moving, then patching the most affected eye may be practical. Otherwise, rest and patch both eyes.

The prescription Tetracaine .5% ophthalmic drops will help ease the pain, but long-term use can delay eye surface healing. Oral pain medication will be of help and should be used. The severe pain can last from hours to several days. In case a drainage of pus or crusting of the eyelids occurs, start antibiotic ophthalmic ointment applications as indicated in the section on conjunctivitis.

CONJUNCTIVITIS

(Infection or inflammation of the eye surface)

An infection of the eye will be heralded by a scratchy feeling, almost indistinguishable from a foreign body in the eye. The sclera (white of the eye) will be reddened. Generally the eye will be matted shut in the morning with pus or granular matter.

Infections are generally caused by bacteria, but viral infections also occur. Viral infections tend to have a blotchy red appearance over the white of the eye, while bacterial infections have a generalized red appearance. The drainage in bacterial infections tends to be pus, while virus usually cause a watery discharge.

Allergic conjunctivitis will result in a faint pink coloration and a clear drainage. There are frequently other symptoms of allergy such as runny nose, no fever, and no lymph node enlargement. With either viral or bacterial conjunctivitis, look for fever and possibly lymph node enlargement in the neck. Runny nose and sinus infection are frequently present also. Be sure that a foreign body is not the cause of the reddish eye and infection. If so, it must be removed.

Rinse with clean water frequently during the day. Eye infections such as common bacterial conjunctivitis, the most common infection, are self-limiting and will generally clear themselves within two weeks. They can become much worse, however, so medical attention should be sought. Do not patch, but protect the eyes from sunlight. When one eye is infected, treat both eyes as the infection spreads easily to the non-infected eye. There is no suitable non-prescription medication, but note the discussion concerning the use of non-Rx Neosporin or Polysporin in the section on eye foreign body removal. From the Rx supplies one could use the Tobrax ophthalmic ointment 3 times a day for 5 to 7 days. Steroids should not be placed in the eye if there is any chance that a viral infection may be present as this could cause severe corneal ulceration. If the infection fails to show improvement within 48 hours, probably the antibiotic will not be effective. Reasons for antibiotic failure include: a missed foreign body, allergy to the antibiotic or to something else such as pollen, or resistance of an infectious germ to the antibiotic being used. Switch medications in the case of no improvement after 48 hours. When no other antibiotic ointment is available, use oral antibiotic such as doxycycline 100 mg, 1 capsule twice daily or the alternative antibiotics suggested for the Rx Oral/Topical Module. If the eye is improving, continue use as indicated above, continuing for a full 24 hours after symptoms have ceased.

IRITIS

Iritis is an inflammatory disease of the eye having the general appearance of conjunctivitis, but while in the latter the reddish color fades to white near the iris of the eye (the colored part), with iritis the rim of sclera (white of the eye) around the iris is more inflamed or reddened than the white portion further out. Protect from sun glare. Give aspirin or other pain medication if available. Have the patient see a physician immediately. The non-Rx treatment will consist of giving the patient ibuprofen 800 mg every 6 hours. Provide sun protection. The prescription treatment would be Lorcet 10/650, 1 tablet every 4 hours. Instill Tobrax ophthalmic ointment three times a day. This patient would benefit from eye dilation and possibly local steroid use under a physician's care.

As iritis progresses, the red blush near the iris will become more pronounced and spasm of muscle used in operation of the iris will cause the pupil to become irregular. With further progression it is possible for the pupil (anterior chamber) to become cloudy, for cataracts and glaucoma to develop, and serious scarring of eye tissues to develop. Sometimes a profound conjunctivitis or corneal abrasion will cause an iritis that will clear as the problem clears. Some cases of mild iritis can be cleared with agents that dilate the pupil without steroid use. All cases of iritis require treatment by an ophthalmologist.

ALLERGIC CONJUNCTIVITIS

The common wilderness causes are sensitivity to inhaled pollens and irritation from wood smoke. This problem is usually associated with a runny nose (rhinitis) and at times swelling of the eyelids. Rarely there will be a generalized skin itching and the appearance of welts (urticaria). In severe cases there can be considerable swelling of the conjunctival covering of the white of the eye (sclera), forming what appears as fluid-filled sacs over the sclera of the eye (but not covering the cornea). This puffy tissue generally has a light pink tinge to it. While this can look terrible, it is not serious and will resolve on its own within 48 hours after further exposure to the causative agent ceases.

From the non-Rx supplies give Actifed 1 tablet 4 times a day and use the tetrahydrozoline eye drops, 2 in each eye every 3 or 4 hours as needed.

STIES AND CHALAZIA

These infections of the eyelid can cause scratching of the cornea surface. Often the victim thinks that something is in the eye when, in fact, one of these small pimples is forming. The sty is an infection along a hair follicle on the eyelid margin. The chalazion is an infection of an oil gland on the inner lid margin. The patient will have redness, pain, and swelling along the edge of the upper or lower eye lid. At times the eye will be red with evidence of infection, or conjunctivitis. An eyelid may be swollen, without the pimple formation, when this problem first develops. There should not be extensive swelling around the eye. That could represent a periorbital cellulitis which is a serious infection requiring treatment with injectable antibiotics. Make sure that a foreign body is not causing the symptoms. Check the eye and eye lids as indicated in that section. While so checking, ascertain if there is a pimple formation that confirms the diagnosis. If it is on the upper lid and it is scratching the eye while blinking, patch the eye and send to a physician for treatment. If no medical care is available, have the patient place warm compresses on the eye for 20 minutes every two hours to cause the sty to come to a head. When it does, it may spontaneously break and drain. If it does not in two days, open it with a flick of a #11 scalpel blade or needle. Continue the warm compresses and provide medication as below. If Rx supplies are available, then instill Tobrax ophthalmic ointment 3 times a day (also note discussion concerning the use of over the counter antibiotic ointment in the eye on page 37). If the lid is quite swollen, give the patient doxycycline 100 mg twice daily or Cefzil 250 mg twice daily. Once localized and draining, the oral antibiotic will not be necessary.

SPONTANEOUS SUBCONJUNCTIVAL HEMORRHAGE

This condition presents as bright bleeding over a portion of the white, or conjunctiva, of the eye. It spreads out over a period of 12 to 48 hours, then reabsorbs slowly over the next 7 to 21 days, next turning the conjunctiva yellowish as the blood is reabsorbed. There should not be any pain with this condition, although some people may report a vague "full" feeling in the eye. It normally occurs without cause, but can appear after blunt trauma, or violent coughing, sneezing, or vomiting. No treatment is necessary.

BLUNT TRAUMA TO THE EYE

The immediate treatment is to immobilize the injured eye as soon as possible by patching both eyes and moving the patient only by litter. Double vision could mean that there has been a fracture of the skull near the eye or that a problem developed within the central nervous system. Double vision is sometimes caused by swelling of tissue behind the eyelid. A hyphema may appear, which is a collection of blood in the anterior chamber of the eye. The blood settles in front of the pupil, behind the cornea, and can settle with a distinct blood fluid level becoming easily noticed simply by looking carefully at the pupil and iris.

Patch as indicated in the section on serious injury eye patch techniques. Patients with hyphema and serious blunt trauma should be evacuated to a physician for care. Have the patient sit with head up, from 45° to 90° to allow blood to pool at the lower edge of the anterior chamber. Check the eye twice daily for drainage which might indicate infection. If infection develops, treat with oral antibiotic such as the doxycycline 100 mg twice daily. The Rx Tobrax ophthalmic ointment may be instilled three times daily. Treat with oral pain medications such as the Rx Lorcet 10/650 one tablet every 4 hours. Give Atarax 25 mg 4 times daily as needed to potentiate the pain medication and help alleviate nausea or 50 mg 4 times daily if required to calm the patient.

Provide the strongest pain medications required to prevent the injured patient from grimacing and squeezing the injured eye, thus possibly compromising the eye contents even more. Small corneal or scleral lacerations may require no treatment at all, but these should be seen and evaluated by a physician if at all possible. It should be noted that severe injury to one eye may even cause blindness to develop in the other eye due to "sympathetic ophthalmia," which is probably an allergic response to eye pigment of the injured eye entering the victim's blood stream.

GLAUCOMA

Glaucoma is the rise of pressure within the eyeball (intraocular pressure increase). The most common form (open angle glaucoma) generally is not encountered before the age of 40. The patient notes halos around lights, mild headaches, loss of vision to the sides (peripheral field cuts), and loss of ability to see well at night. The external eye usually appears normal. This frequently affects both eyes. This condition is generally of gradual onset so that the patient can consult a physician upon returning from the bush.

Initial treatment is with a prescription drug, one drop of 0.5% pilocarpine. It would not be necessary to carry this particular medication, except to treat this condition. This problem should be detected by the pretrip physical examination. Everyone over the age of 40 should have their intraocular pressure tested prior to departure.

Acute glaucoma (narrow angle glaucoma) is much less common than open angle glaucoma, but is much more spectacular in onset. Acute glaucoma is characterized by a rapid rise in pressure of the fluid within the eyeball causing blurred vision, severe pain in the eye, and even abdominal distress from vagal nerve stimulation. An acute attack can sometimes be broken with pilocarpine, but often needs emergency surgery. A thorough eye examination should be done before the trip to discover those eyes with narrow angles that could result in acute glaucoma. In eyes likely to develop acute glaucoma, a laser iridectomy can be done as an outpatient to prevent an acute narrow angle glaucoma attack.

Events that might precipitate an acute glaucoma attack can include the use of certain medications, such as decongestants. If anyone develops severe eye pain while taking a decongestant or other non-essential medication, have them stop taking it immediately. Severe eye pain from any cause is a reason for urgent evacuation of the patient.

NOSE PROBLEMS

NASAL CONGESTION

Nasal congestion is caused by an allergic reaction to pollen, dust, or other allergens, and viral or bacterial upper respiratory infections. Bacterial infections can be cured with antibiotics, but otherwise all are treated similarly for symptomatic relief. Use Actifed, which should be taken 1 tablet every 6 hours as needed for nasal congestion. Treat for discomfort with Percogesic from the non-Rx supplies as needed. Drink lots of liquid to prevent the mucus from becoming too thick. Thick mucus will not drain well and this tends to allow it to pack the sinus cavities with increasingly painful pressure.

If the patient has no fever, do not give an antibiotic. A low grade temperature is probably viral and still does not warrant an antibiotic. If a temperature greater than 101° F (38° C) is present, then treat with antibiotic such as the doxycycline 100 mg twice daily or the Cefzil 250 mg twice daily from the Rx supplies.

FOREIGN BODY, NOSE

Foul drainage from one nostril is very suspicious of a foreign body. In adults the history of something being placed up the nose would, of course, help in the diagnosis. In a child drainage from one nostril must be considered to be a foreign body until ruled out. Have the patient try to blow his nose to remove the foreign body. With an infant it may be possible for a parent to gently puff into the baby's mouth to force the object out of the nose. While having a nasal speculum would be ideal, using the Field Surgical Module one can improvise by using the mosquito or Hartman hemostats (see page 209). Spread the tips apart after placing them just inside the nostril. One can stretch the nostril quite extensively without causing pain. Shine a light into the nostril passage and attempt to spot the foreign body. Try to grasp the object with another forceps or other instrument under direct visualization in this manner. If the foreign material is loose debris, say a capsule that broke in the patient's mouth and which was sneezed into the nostrils, it is best to irrigate this material out rather than attempting to cleanse with a Q-tip, etc. Place a bulb or irrigation syringe in the clear nostril. With the patient repeating an "eng" sound, flush water and hopefully the debris out the opposite nostril.

After removing a foreign body, be sure to check the nostril again for an additional one. Try not to push a foreign body down the back of the patient's throat where they may choke on it. If this is unavoidable, have the patient face down and bend over to decrease the chance of choking. After pushing the object further into the nose and into the upper part of the pharynx, hopefully the victim can cough the object out. If you are using this technique, first read the sections on nose bleed and the Heimlich maneuver.

NOSE BLEED

(Epistaxis)

If nose bleeding is caused from a contusion to the nose, the bleeding is usually self limited. Bleeding that starts without trauma is generally more difficult to stop. Most bleeding is from small arteries located near the front of the nose partition, or nasal septum. The best treatment is direct pressure. Have the victim squeeze the nose between her fingers for ten minutes by the clock (a very long time when there is no clock to watch). If this fails, squeeze another ten minutes. Do not blow the nose for this will dislodge clots and start the bleeding all over again. If the bleeding is severe, have the victim sit up to prevent choking on blood and to aid in the reduction of the blood pressure in the nose. Cold compresses do little good.

Continued bleeding can result in shock. This will in turn decrease the bleeding. The sitting position is mandatory to prevent choking on blood from a severe bleed and, as indicated above, will aid in the reduction of blood pressure in the nose. Taken to the extreme degree this position aids in allowing shock to occur.

Another technique that can be tried is to wet a gauze strip thoroughly with the epinephrine from the syringe in the Anakit or AnaGuard, a component of the prescription medical kit. The epinephrine can act as a vasoconstrictor to decrease the blood flow and allow clotting. Those having only non-prescription medical supplies will have to use the tetrahydrozoline eye drops, which will not be as powerful in their action. First, clear the nose of blood clot so the gauze can be in direct contact with the nasal membranes. Have the victim blow their nose or use the irrigation syringe. Place the epinephrine soaked gauze in the nose and apply pinching pressure. Pinch for ten minute increments. The gauze may be removed after the bleeding has stopped.

NOSE FRACTURE

(Broken Nose)

A direct blow causing a nasal fracture is associated with pain, swelling, and nasal bleeding. The pain is usually point tender, which means that a very light touch elicits pain, indicating that a fracture has occurred at that location. While the bleeding from trauma to the nose can initially be intense, it seldom lasts more than a few minutes. Apply a cold compress, if available. Allow the patient to pinch their nose to aid in reducing bleeding.

If the nose is laterally displaced (shoved to one side), push it back into place. More of these fractures have been treated by coaches on the playing field than have been reduced by doctors. If it is a depressed fracture, a specialist will have to properly elevate the fragments. As soon as the person returns from the bush, have him seen by a physician, but this is not a reason for expensive urgent evacuation. Provide pain medication, but this should only be necessary for a few doses. It is rare to need to pack a bleeding nose due to trauma and this should be avoided, if possible, due to the increased pain it would cause.

THE EAR

Problems with the ear involve pain, loss of hearing, or drainage. Traumas involving the ear could include lacerations, blunt trauma and hemorrhage (bleeding) in the outer ear tissue, damage from pressure changes of the ear drum (barotrauma) from diving, high altitude, explosions or direct blows to the ear.

TABLE 2

SYMPTOMS AND SIGNS OF EAR PATHOLOGY

	Hearing Loss	Pain	Head Congestion	Ear Drainage	Fever
Trauma *(Page 53)*	xx	xx		x	
Foreign Body *(Page 52)*		x		x	
Infection					
inner ear *(Page 50)*	xx	xx	xx	*	xx
outer ear *(Page 51)*	x	xx		x	x
Allergy *(Page 49)*	x	x	xx		
Dental Source *(Page 58)*		x			
TMJ Source *(Page 53)*		x			
Lymph Node Source *(Page 50)*		x			

xx = A frequent or intense symptom
x = Common, less intense symptom
Blank = Less likely to produce this symptom

* only if the ear drum ruptures will drainage occur in an inner ear infection, but at that moment the pain decreases remarkably.

EARACHE

Pain in the ear can be associated with a number of sources, as indicated in Table 2. The history of trauma will be an obvious source of pain as mentioned. Most ear pain is due to an *otitis media* or infection behind the ear drum (tympanic membrane), *otitis externa* or infection in the outer ear canal (auditory canal), or due to infection elsewhere (generally a dental infection, infected tonsil, or lymph node in the neck near the ear). Allergy can result in pressure behind the ear drum and is also a common source of ear pain.

In the bush a simple physical examination and the additional medical history will readily (and generally accurately) distinguish the difference between an otitis media or otitis externa, and sources of pain beyond the ear. Pushing on the nob at the front of the ear (the tragus) or pulling on the ear lobe will elicit pain with an otitis externa. This will not hurt if the patient has otitis media. The history of head congestion also favors otitis media. A swollen tender nodule in the neck near the ear would be an infected lymph node. If the skin above the swelling is red, the patient probably has an infected skin abscess. The pain from an abscess is so localized, that confusion with an ear infection is seldom a problem. (Refer to section on abscess, page 57). One or more tender lymph nodes can hurt to the extent that confusion of the exact source of the pain may be in doubt. Swollen, tender lymph nodes in the neck are usually associated with pharyngitis (sore throat), with severe otitis externa, or with infections of the skin in the scalp. The latter should be readily noted by examination - palpate the scalp for infected cysts or abscesses. Dental caries, or cavities, can hurt to the extent that the pain seems to come from the ear. They can ordinarily be identified during a careful examination of the mouth. If an obvious cavity is not visualized with a light, try tapping on each tooth to see if pain is suddenly elicited. (Refer to dental caries, page 58).

OTITIS EXTERNA

(Outer Ear Infection)

This infection of the auditory canal is commonly called "swimmer's ear". The external auditory canal generally becomes inflamed from conditions of high humidity, accumulation of ear wax, or contact with contaminated water. Scratching the ear after picking the nose or scratching elsewhere may also be a source of this common infection.

Prevent cold air from blowing against the ear. Warm packs against the ear or instilling comfortably warm sweet oil or even cooking oil can help. Provide pain medication. Obtain professional help if the patient develops a fever, the pain becomes severe, or lymph nodes or adjacent neck tissues start swelling. Significant tissue swelling will require antibiotic treatment. At times a topical ointment will suffice, but with fever, swollen lymph or skin structures an oral antibiotic will be required.

Triple antibiotic or Polysporin antibiotic ointment available without a prescription will work fine for outer ear infections. This is not approved by the FDA for this use, as ear infections are serious and it is not intended that non-physicians treat this condition without medical help. From the Rx kit, one should use the Tobrax ophthalmic (eye) ointment. Any of the above ointments should be applied with the ear facing up and allowed to melt by body temperature. This may take 5 minutes per ear. Place cotton in the ear to hold the medication in place. Instill ointment 4 times daily and treat for

14 days. If the canal is swollen shut, a steroid ointment may also be used in between applications of the other ointments just described. From the non-Rx Topical Bandaging Module use the hydrocortisone 1% cream, or from the Rx Oral/Topical Medication Module use Topicort .25% cream. Swollen tissue and/or fever also means that an oral antibiotic is required. From the Rx Oral/Topical Medication Module use the doxycycline 100 mg twice daily or the Cefzil 250 mg twice daily. Provide the best pain medication that you can, from your non-Rx Oral Medication Module use 1 or 2 Percogesic every four hours. From the Rx Oral/Topical Medication Module give Lorcet 10/650, 1 tablet every 4 hours as needed.

OTITIS MEDIA

(Middle Ear Infection)

This condition will present in a person who has sinus congestion and possibly drainage from allergy or infection. The ear pain can be excruciating. Fever will frequently be intermittent, normal at one moment and over 103° F (39° C) at other times. Fever indicates bacterial infection of the fluid trapped behind the ear drum. If the ear drum ruptures, the pain will cease immediately and the fever will drop. This drainage allows the body to cure the infection, but will result in at least temporary damage to the ear drum and decreased hearing until it heals. There is no pain when pulling on the ear lobe or pushing on the tragus with this condition, unless an outer ear infection is also present. If you were to look at the ear drum with an otoscope, it would be red and bulging out from pressure or sucked back by a vacuum in the middle ear.

You do not need an otoscope to diagnose this condition. Many people will complain of hearing loss and think they have wax or a foreign body in the ear canal, when they actually have fluid accumulation behind the ear drum. Ear drops and washing the ear will not help improve this condition. Besides pain, the key to the diagnosis is head congestion and fever. There is little that can be accomplished without medication. Protect the ear from cold, position the head so that the ear is directed upwards, and provide warm packs to the ear. While drops do not help cure this problem, some pain relief may be obtained with warmed sweet oil (or even cooking oil) drops in the ear.

Treatment will consist of providing decongestant, pain medication and oral antibiotic. A good decongestant is Actifed, 1 tablet 4 times daily. The pain medication is given as needed as indicated in the previous section.

Only the Rx Oral/Topical Module has the proper antibiotics to treat this condition. Use doxycycline 1 tablet twice daily or Cefzil 250 mg twice daily, generally for 5 to 7 days.

If the pressure causes the ear drum to rupture, the pain and fever will cease, but there will be a bloody drainage from the ear. Hearing is always decreased with the infection and will remained decreased due to the ruptured ear drum for some time. This generally heals itself quite well, but treat with decongestant to decrease the drainage and allow the ear drum to heal. Avoid placing drops or ointments in the ear canal if there is a chance that the ear drum has ruptured, as many medications are damaging to the inner ear mechanisms.

FOREIGN BODY, EAR

These are generally of three types. Accumulation of wax plugs (cerumen), foreign objects, and living insects. Wax plugs can usually be softened with a warmed oil. This may have to be placed in the ear canal repeatedly over many days. Irrigating with room temperature water may be attempted with a bulb syringe, such as the one recommended for wound irrigation in the Field Surgical Module. If a wax plugged ear becomes painful, treat as indicated in the section on otitis externa.

The danger in trying to remove inanimate objects is the tendency to shove them further into the ear canal or to damage the delicate ear canal lining, thus adding bleeding to your troubles. Of course, rupturing the ear drum by shoving against it would be a real unnecessary disaster. Attempt to grasp a foreign body with a pair of tweezers if you can visualize it. Do not poke blindly with anything. Irrigation may be attempted as indicated above. A popular method of aiding in the management of insects in the ear canal is the instillation of lidocaine to kill the bug instantly prior to attempting removal. There are reports of lidocaine making a person very dizzy, especially if it leaks through a hole in the ear drum into the inner ear. This dizziness is very distressing if it happens and results in profound vomiting and discomfort should it occur. It is self limiting and should not last more than a day if it does transpire. An alternate method is to drown the bug with cooking or other oil, then attempt removal. Oil seems to kill bugs quicker than water. The less struggle, the less chance for stinging, biting, or other trauma to the delicate ear canal and ear drum. Tilt the ear downward, thus hoping to slide the dead bug towards the entrance where it can be grappled. Shinning a light at the ear to coax a bug out is probably futile.

RUPTURED EAR DRUM

(Tympanic Membrane Perforation)

Rupture of the ear drum can result from direct puncture, from explosions, and from the barotrauma of diving deep or rapid ascent to high altitude. Being smacked on the ear can also rupture the ear drum.

Avoid diving or rapid ascents of altitude in vehicles or airplanes if suffering from sinus congestion. Congestion can lead to blockage of the eustachian tube. Failure to equilibrate pressure through this tube between the middle ear and the throat - and thus the outside world - can result in damage to the ear drum. In case of congestion, take a decongestant such as Actifed 1 tablet every 4 hours until clear. Cancel any plans of diving if congested. Also, if a gradual pressure squeeze is causing pain while diving, the dive should be terminated.

When flying, it will be noted that blocked eustachian tubes will cause more pain upon descent than ascent. When going up the pressure in the inner ear will increase and blow out through the eustachian tube. When coming down increased outer atmospheric pressure is much less apt to clear the plugged tube and a squeeze of air against the ear drum will result. Try to equalize this pressure by pinching the nose shut and gently increasing the pressure in your mouth and throat against closed lips. This will generally clear the eustachian tube and relieve the air squeeze on the ear drum. Do not overdo this; that can also be painful. If barotrauma results in ear drum rupture, the pain should instantly cease. There may be bloody drainage from the ear canal. Do not place drops in the ear canal. Drainage can be gently wiped away or frequently changed cotton plugs used to catch the bloody fluid.

TMJ SYNDROME

This is actually a problem of the jaw, but the pain radiates into the ear so often, that we will consider it primarily as a source of ear pain. The temporal-mandibular joint is the hinge joint of the jaw, located just forward of the ear. You can easily feel it move if you place a finger tip into your ear canal. When this joint becomes inflamed, it will frequently cause ear pain. It will then be painful to finger tip pressure directly on the joint. No swelling should be noted. Tenderness is increased with chewing, and pain and popping or locking may be noted when opening the jaw widely.

Treatment is with local heat. The use of ibuprofen or Percogesic can be very helpful. At times Lorcet 10/650, 1 tablet every 4 hours, may be required. Do not eat foods that are hard to chew or which require opening the mouth widely.

THE MOUTH AND THROAT

SORE THROAT

(Pharyngitis)

The most common cause of a sore throat, or pharyngitis, is a viral infection. While uncomfortable, this malady requires no antibiotic treatment - in fact, antibiotics will do no good whatsoever. Strictly speaking, the only sore throat that needs to be treated is the one caused by a specific bacteria (beta hemolytic streptococcus, Lancefield group A) as it has been found that treatment for 10 days will avoid the dreaded complication of rheumatic fever which may occur in 1 to 3 percent of the people who contract this particular infection. Many purists in the medical profession feel that no antibiotics should be used until the results of a throat culture or antibody screen proving this particular infection have been returned from the lab. On a short trip the victim can be taken to a doctor for a strep culture to determine if the sore throat was indeed strep. On a wilderness trip longer than 2 weeks, it would be best to commit the patient to a 10 day therapy of antibiotic, realizing that the symptoms will soon pass and the patient may seem well, but that it is essential to continue the medication for 10 days.

There are text book differences in the general appearance of a viral and strep sore throat. The lymph nodes in the neck are swollen in both cases, they are more tender with bacterial infections, but people with a low pain threshold will complain bitterly about soreness regardless of the source of infection. The throat will be quite red in bacterial infection and a white splotchy coating over the red tonsils or back portion of the throat generally means a strep infection - at least these classic indications are present 20 percent of the time. Sore throats caused by some viral infections (namely infectious mononucleosis and adenovirus) may mimic all of the above. From the Rx Oral/Topical Medication Module use Cefzil 250 mg twice daily for 10 days.

INFECTIOUS MONONUCLEOSIS

This disease of young adults (teens through 30 years of age), generally presents as a terrible sore throat, swollen lymph nodes (normally at the back of the neck and not as tender as with strep infection), and a profound tired feeling. It is self-limited with total recovery to be expected after 2 weeks for most victims - some, unfortunately are bedridden for weeks and lethargic for 6 months. Spleen enlargement is common. The most serious aspect of this disease is the possibility of splenic rupture, but this is rare. Avoid palpating the spleen (shoving on the left upper quadrant of the abdomen), let the victim rest, no hiking, etc., until the illness and feeling of lethargy has passed. The first 5 days are the worst, with fever and excruciating sore throat being the major complaint.

Treatment is symptomatic with medication for fever and pain such as the Non-Rx Percogesic 1 or 2 tablets every 4 to 6 hours, or the Rx Lorcet 10/650 1 tablet every 4 to 6 hours. A mild form of hepatitis frequently occurs with mononucleosis that causes nausea and loss of appetite. This requires no specific treatment other than rest. If severe ear pain begins, add a decongestant such as Actifed 1 tablet every 6 hours to promote relief of eustachian tube pressure. Due to the uncertainty of diagnosis, treat the severe sore throat as if it were a strep infection with antibiotic for 10 days as indicated above.

MOUTH SORES

When these develop the two concerns that the patient frequently has is the possibility of cancer or infection, especially herpes. A common reason for a lesion is the sore called a papilloma caused from rubbing against a sharp tooth or dental work. They can look serious, but are not. They are raised, normally orange in color. Usually one can find an obvious rough area causing the irritation. Treatment is to avoid chewing at the lesion, apply eugenol or other anesthetic agent, or from the Rx Oral/Topical Medication Module, Kenalog in orabase every 3 hours.

A canker sore, also called an aphthous ulcer, can appear anywhere in the mouth and be any size. It has a distinctive appearance of a white crater with a red, swollen border. Treatment is as above.

If there is generalized tissue swelling, possibly drainage or whitish cover on the gums, the breath is foul smelling and the gums and tissue of the mouth bleed easily when scraped, it is possible that the victim has trench mouth or Vincent's infection. This is caused by poor hygiene, which is unfortunately common on long expeditions under adverse circumstances. If the white exudate is located over the tonsils, one has to be concerned about strep throat (see page 54), mononucleosis (see page 54), and diphtheria. Treat trench mouth with warm water rinses, swishing the crude off as well as possible. If the Rx Oral/Topical Medication Module is available, give Cefzil 250 mg twice daily for 4 to 5 days.

The mouth lesions of herpes simplex begin as small blisters that leave a raw area once they have broken open. The ulceration from a herpes is red rather than the white of the canker sore. They are very painful. While Zovirax is the Rx drug of choice, application of topical anesthetic such as the Non-Rx dibucaine ointment will provide pain relief for the 10 days or so that the lesions are active. Application of the Rx Kenalog in orabase relieves the inflammation rapidly. Zovirax has not been recommended for inclusion in the Wilderness Medical Kit modules, but if you are bothered with this problem frequently, consider doing so.

Fever blisters are sores that break out on the vermillion border of the lips, generally as a result of herpes simplex virus eruptions. These lesions can be activated by fevers (hence their name "fever blister"), or other trauma, even mental stress. Ultra violet light will frequently cause flares of fever blisters. This can be a common problem of mountain travel due to the more intense UV radiation encountered at higher altitudes. Treat as above for the herpes simplex inner mouth lesions. These lesions can be prevented with adequate sunscreen (generally a total block such as zinc oxide ointment is required) or by taking Zovirax capsules, 400 mg twice daily.

GUM PAIN OR SWELLING

Pain attended by swelling high on the gum at the base of the tooth, usually indicates an infection and a tooth that may require extraction, or root canal therapy, if a dentist can be consulted who has brought more than just his fly rod with him on the trip. Attempting to treat without either option, have the patient use warm water mouth rinses. Start the victim on antibiotics as indicated in the previous section. If a bulging area can be identified in the mouth, an incision into the swollen gum with a #11 scalpel blade may promote drainage. If the pain is severe and not relieved with the Rx Lorcet 10/650, or any other pain medication which you have, the tooth may have to be pulled.

Swelling at the gum line, rather than at the base of the tooth, may indicate a periodontal abscess. The gingiva (or gums) are red, swollen, foul smelling and oozing. Frequently this represents food particle entrapment and abscess formation along the surface of the tooth with the gums - the so-called gingival cuff. Considerable relief can often be obtained by probing directly into the abscess area through the gingival cuff, using any thin, blunt instrument. Probe along the length of the tooth to break up and drain the abscess. Have the patient use frequent hot mouth rinses to continue the drainage process. If a foreign object, such as a piece of food, is causing the swelling, irrigate with warm salt solution or warm water, with sufficient force to dislodge the particle. Probe it loose if necessary. Dental floss may be very helpful.

Acute pain and swelling of the tissue behind the third molar usually represents an erupting wisdom tooth. Technically this is called "pericoronitis." There is a little flap of tissue that lies over the erupting wisdom tooth called the "operculum." Biting on this causes it to swell, and then it becomes much easier to bite on it again, and so on... The end result is considerable pain. This can be relieved by surgically removing the operculum. If local anesthetic is available, such as lidocaine, inject it directly into the operculum and then cut it out with a scalpel blade using the outline of the erupting tooth as a guideline. The bleeding can soon be stopped by biting down on a gauze or other cloth after the procedure is over. Stitching this wound is not required. If no lidocaine is available, swab the area with alcohol as this helps provide some slight anesthesia. Application of topical anesthetic, such as the non-Rx 1% dibucaine or the Rx Tetracaine .5% ophthalmic drops, may also be of slight help.

Swelling of the entire side of the face will occur with dental infections that spread. This condition should ideally be treated in a hospital with intravenous antibiotics. In the bush, apply warm compresses to the face. Do not lance these from the skin side, but a peaked, bulging area on the inside of the mouth may be lanced to promote drainage. Abscess extension into surrounding facial tissues generally means that lancing will do little good. This patient is very ill and rest is mandatory. Provide antibiotic coverage from the Rx Oral/Topical Medication Module with Cefzil 250 mg 2 capsules every 12 hours or from the Rx Injectable Module Rocephin 500 mg intramuscular injection every 12 hours.

MOUTH LACERATIONS

Any significant trauma to the mouth causes considerable bleeding and concern. The bleeding initially always seems worse than it is. Rinse the mouth with warm water to clear away the clots so that you can tell where the bleeding has been coming from.

Laceration of the piece of tissue that seems to join the bottom lip or upper lip to the gum line is a common result of trauma to the mouth and need not be repaired, even though it initially looks horrible and may bleed considerably. This is called the labial frenum. Simply stuff some gauze into the area until the bleeding stops.

A laceration of the tongue will not require stitching (suturing) unless an edge is deeply involved. Fairly deep cuts along the top surface and bottom can be ignored in the wilderness setting. If suturing is to be accomplished and you have injectable lidocaine from the Rx Injectable Module, inject into the lower gum behind the teeth on the side of the gum facing the tongue. Technically this area is called the median raphe distal to the posterior teeth. This will block the side of the tongue and be much less painful than directly injecting into the tongue. Use the 3-0 gut sutures. These sutures will dissolve within a few days. Sutures in the tongue frequently come out within a few hours, even when they are well tied, much to the victim and surgeon's annoyance. If this happens and the tongue is not bleeding badly, just leave it alone. Minor cuts along the edge of the tongue can also be ignored.

Make sure that cuts on the inside of the mouth do not have foreign bodies, such as pieces of tooth inside of them. These must be removed. Inject the lidocaine into the wound before probing if you have the Rx Injectable Medication Module. Irrigate thoroughly with water. Even without the lidocaine, the inside of the mouth can be stitched with minimal pain. Use the 3-0 gut suture, removing them in 4 days if the suture has not fallen out already. Refer to page 95 for discussion of suturing the face and the outside portion of the lips.

DENTAL PAIN

Cavities may be identified by visual examination of the mouth in most cases. At times the pain is so severe that the patient cannot tell exactly which tooth is the offender. A painful tooth will not refer pain to the opposite side of the mouth. Painful back teeth normally do not refer pain to front teeth and vice-versa. With the painful area narrowed down, look for an obvious cavity. If none is found, tap each tooth in turn until the offending one is reached; a tap on it will elicit strong pain.

Dry the tooth and try to clean out any cavity found. For years oil of cloves, or eugenol, has been used to deaden dental pain. Avoid trying to apply an aspirin directly to a painful tooth, it will only make a worse mess of things. Many excellent dental kits are now available without prescription that contain topical anesthetic agents and temporary fillings. A daub of topical anesthetic such as the 1% dibucaine ointment will work. Before applying the anesthetic, dry the tooth and try to clean out any cavity found. From the Rx kit, Lorcet 10/650 1 tab every 4 hours will generally eliminate the most severe dental pain, or from the non-Rx kit, give Percogesic 2 tabs every 4 hours for pain. When in the bush and a toothache begins, I would also start treating with an antibiotic if the Rx kit is available. Give Cefzil 250 mg 2 caps twice daily for 2 days, then 1 capsule twice daily until any swelling or pain resolves.

LOST FILLING

This could turn into a real disaster. An old fashioned remedy was to use powdered zinc oxide (not the ointment) and eugenol. Starting with the two in equal parts, mix until a putty is formed by adding more zinc oxide powder as necessary. This always takes considerably more of the zinc oxide than at first would seem necessary. Pack this putty into the cavity and allow to set over the next 24 hours.

The Cavit dental filling paste in the Rx Oral/Topical Unit provides a strong temporary filling. Dry the cavity bed thoroughly with a gauze square. Place several drops of anesthetic, such as the oil of cloves (eugenol), to deaden the nerve endings and kill bacteria. Dibucaine ointment from the Non-Rx Oral/Topical Module can be used for this purpose. You will have to pack the ointment into the cavity area and allow it to melt. Dry the cavity carefully once again. The Cavit paste should be applied to the dry cavity and packed firmly into place. Obviously avoid biting on the side of the filling, regardless of the materials used to make your temporary filling. See a dentist as soon as possible as the loss of a filling may indicate extension of decay in the underlying tooth.

LOOSE OR DISLODGED TOOTH

When you examine a traumatized mouth and find a tooth that is rotated, or dislocated in any direction, do not push the tooth back into place. Further movement may disrupt the tooth's blood and nerve supply. If the tooth is at all secure leave it alone. The musculature of the lips and tongue will generally gently push the tooth back into place and keep it there.

A fractured tooth with exposed pink substance that is bleeding, is showing exposed nerve. This tooth will need protection with eugenol and temporary filling as indicated above. This is actually a dental emergency that should be treated by a dentist immediately.

If a tooth is knocked out, replace it into the socket immediately. If this cannot be done, have the victim hold the tooth under their tongue or in their lower lip until it can be implanted. In any case, hours are a matter of great importance. A tooth left out too long will be rejected by the body as a foreign substance.

All of the above problems will mean that a soft diet and avoidance of chewing with the affected tooth for many days will be necessary. In the wilderness setting, start the patient on antibiotic such as the doxycycline 100 mg, 1 daily for any of the above problems.

Trauma that can cause any of the above may also result in fractures of the tooth below the gum line and of the alveolar ridge affecting several teeth. If this is suspected, start the patient on antibiotic as mentioned in the paragraph above. Oral surgical help must be obtained as soon as possible. A soft diet is essential until healing takes place, possibly a matter of 6 to 8 weeks.

PULLING A TOOTH

It is best not to pull a tooth from an infected gum as this might spread the infection. If an abscess is forming, place the patient on antibiotic, such as the Cefzil 250 mg twice daily or the doxycycline 100 mg twice daily, and use warm mouth rinses to promote drainage. After the infection has subsided it will be safer to pull the tooth. Opening the abscess as described in the paragraph on dental abscess on page 57 will be helpful at times. If it appears necessary to pull an infected tooth, give the patient an antibiotic pill about 2 hours before pulling the tooth to provide some protection against spreading the infection. Pull the tooth by obtaining a secure hold with the universal side cutting rongeur (Figure 6). Slowly apply pressure in a back-and-forth, side-to-side motion to rock the tooth free. This loosens the tooth in its socket and will permit its removal.

Avoid jerking or pulling the tooth with a straight outward force; it can resist all of the strength that you have in this direction. Jerking may break off the root. The rongeur will grip the tooth surface by cutting into the enamel, holding better than even dental extraction forceps

If the root breaks off, you may leave it alone rather than trying to dig it out. If

FIGURE 6. *The side cutting dental rongeur used as an universal tooth extractor.*

the root section is obviously loose, then you can pick it out with some suitable instrument. Thin fragments of bone may fracture off during the extraction. These will work their way to the surface during healing. Do not attempt to replace them, but pick them free as they surface.

If you do not have dental forceps, it is best to not attempt to pull the tooth with another instrument. Pliers may crush the tooth and the tooth will slip in your grasp. Even a large, solid tooth can be removed by using your finger to rock it back and forth. This may take days to accomplish, but it will eventually loosen sufficiently to remove.

CHEST

One of the most common reasons for a visit to a physician's office or Emergency Department, is a problem with the chest. Chest pain and shortness of breath can be symptoms of serious disorders and cannot be taken lightly. Fortunately, most times the chest pain is benign, generally due to muscle spasm. It can be very difficult to evaluate, even at the Emergency Department. Chest problems are best evaluated by a physician, but in a remote area, try to sort out your options with the table on page 18.

PNEUMONIA—BRONCHITIS
Infection of the airways in the lung (bronchitis) or infection in the air sacks of the lung (pneumonia) will cause very high fever, persistent cough frequently producing phlegm stained with blood, and cause prostration of the victim. From the non-Rx Oral Medication Module treat the fever with Percogesic 2 tablets every 4 hours or ibuprofen 200 mg 2 tablets every 4 hours and the cough with Benadryl 25 mg every 4 hours (see page 206). If you have the Rx Oral/Topical Medication Module you may treat sharp pleuritic chest pain with Lorcet 10/650, 1 tablet every 4 to 6 hours. It is also a strong cough suppressor as mentioned on page 212. Cool with a wet cloth over the forehead as needed. Do not bundle the patient with a very high fever as this will drive the temperature only higher. The shivering cold feeling that the patient has is only proof that his thermal control mechanism is out of adjustment. Trust the thermometer or the back of your hand to follow the patient's temperature. Encourage the patient to drink fluids, as fever and coughing lead to dehydration. This causes the mucus in the bronchioles to become thick and tenacious. Force fluid to prevent this sputum from plugging up sections of the lung.

Provide antibiotic. From the Rx Oral/Topical Medication Module give the Cefzil 250 mg 2 capsules every 12 hours until the fever is broken and then 1 capsule every 12 hours for an additional four days. Or, from the Rx Injectable Module you may give Rocephin 500 mg twice daily. Prepare a sheltered camp for the victim as best as circumstances permit. Rest until the fever is broken is essential with or without the availability of antibiotic. Even though very ill people lose their appetite, encourage the patient to eat.

PULMONARY EMBOLUS

A pulmonary embolus is a blood clot breaking loose from its point of origin, normally from a leg or pelvic vein, which then lodges in the lung after passing through the heart. When serious this condition presents as shortness of breath, rapid breathing, with a dull substernal chest pain. There may be cough, bloody sputum, fever, and sharp chest pain. A pulmonary embolus can mimic pneumonia (page 61) and high altitude pulmonary edema (page 196). It can be fatal if an embolus large enough to block off more than 50 percent of the lung circulation occurs at once. This condition generally resolves within a matter of days. Increased risk is found in older people who have been sitting a long time (such as on plane flights) or anyone immobilized after injury. The only medication in the suggested wilderness medical kit that would be of any help would be the ibuprofen 200 mg given 4 times daily. Stronger doses of this product or additional pain medication can be given to help with the discomfort. Due to the uncertainty of the diagnosis, treat with antibiotic, Cefzil 250 mg 2 capsules twice daily until the pain and/or fever resolves and then 1 capsule twice daily for an additional 4 days. This would not help a pulmonary embolus, but it would properly treat a pneumonia.

THE ABDOMEN

Even with years of clinical experience and unlimited laboratory and x-ray facilities, abdominal pain can be a diagnostic dilemma. How serious is it? Should the trip be terminated and evacuation started or can it be waited out or safely treated in the bush? Or what treatment protocol can be followed by those travelers in isolated areas where there is no chance of rescue?

Any abdominal pain which lasts longer than 24 hours is a cause for concern and professional help should be sought if possible. Diagnosis will be determined from the history (type and severity of pain, location, radiation, when it started) as well as certain aspects of the physical examination and the clinical course that develops. Some of these aspects are summarized in Table 3 and in the discussion which follows.

TABLE 3					
SYMPTOMS AND SIGNS OF ABDOMINAL PATHOLOGY					
	Burning	Nausea*	Food Related	Diarrhea	Fever
Gastritis/ulcer *(page 63)*	xx	x	xx		
Pancreatitis *(page 63)*	xx	x	x		x
Hiatal Hernia *(page 64)*	xx		x		
Gallbladder *(page 64)*		xx	xx		x
Appendicitis *(page 65)*		x			x
Gastroenteritis *(page 66)*		xx	x	xx	x
Diverticulitis *(page 68)*			x	x	x
Colitis *(page 68)*				xx	
Hepatitis *(page 168)*		xx	x		x
Food Poisoning *(page 82)*		xx	xx	xx	x

xx = A frequent or intense symptom
x = Common, less intense symptom
Blank = Less likely to produce this symptom
* See also section on nausea and vomiting, page 67

A burning sensation in the middle of the upper part of the abdomen (mid-epigastrium) is probably GASTRITIS. If allowed to persist this can develop into an ULCER, which is a crater eaten into the stomach or duodenal wall. In the latter case the pain may be most notable in the right upper quadrant. For some reason ulcers will sometimes feel better if you press against them with your hand. This supposedly was why Napoleon is seen with his hand inside his jacket in his favorite pose—he was pressing against his abdomen to relieve the pain of an ulcer. Severe, persistent mid-epigastric pain, that is also frequently burning in nature, can be PANCREATITIS.

This is a serious problem, but rare. Alcohol consumption can cause pancreatitis, as well as gastritis and ulcer formation. It must be avoided if pain in this area develops. In fact, any food that seems to increase the symptoms should be avoided. Reflux of stomach acid up the esophagus, caused by a HIATAL HERNIA, will cause the same symptoms. The reflux also causes the burning pain to radiate up the center of the chest.

Treatment for all of the above is aggressive antacid therapy. These conditions can be made worse by eating spicy food, tomato products, and other foods high in acid content. Avoid any medications containing aspirin and ibuprofen. Acid suppression medication such as Tagamet, Zantac, Pepcid, Axid, and Prilosec help greatly and consideration should be given to adding them to the medical kit for anyone with a history of these disorders. There is a concern that these medications can make the user more vulnerable to traveler's diarrhea, cholera, and other infectious disease from which a normal or high stomach acid level might otherwise provide some protection. A safer medication for persons afflicted with heartburn not responsive to antacids, who must travel in a third world situation, would be Carafate taken 1 gram 4 times daily. This is a prescription medication.

Mild nausea may be associated with the above problems, but intense nausea should make you suspicious of gastroenteritis and food poisoning (generally these cause significant diarrhea also), hepatitis, and gallbladder disorder.

GASTROENTERITIS, see page 66

HEPATITIS, see page 168

Nausea associated with pain in the right upper quadrant of the abdomen may be from a GALLBLADDER problem. There is no burning associated with gallbladder pain. This discomfort is typically made worse by eating, sometimes even smelling, greasy foods. While drinking cream or milk would initially help the pain of gastritis or an ulcer, it would cause an immediate increase in symptoms if the gallbladder is involved. Treatment is avoidance of fatty foods. Nausea and vomiting can be treated as indicated on page 67. Treat for pain as described on page 30. The onset of fever is an important indication of infection of the blocked gallbladder. This is a surgical emergency. Treat with the strongest antibiotic available. If the Rx Injectable Module is available, give Rocephin 500 mg, 2 doses IM immediately, repeated with 2 doses every 12 hours. Lacking that medication, give the Floxin 400 mg every 12 hours. Continue to treat the pain and nausea as required for relief. Offer as much fluid as they can tolerate. Gallbladder disease is more common in overweight people over the age of thirty. It is more common in women.

The possibility of APPENDICITIS is a major concern as it can occur in any age group, and that includes healthy wilderness travelers. It is fortunately rare. While surgery is the treatment of choice, probably as many as 70% of people not treated with surgery or antibiotics can survive this problem. The survival rate would be much higher with appropriate IV therapy. Of course, timely surgery provides 100% survival.

The classic presentation of this illness is a vague feeling of discomfort around the umbilicus (navel). Temperature may be below grade, 99.6 to 100° F (37° C) at first. Within a matter of 12 hours the discomfort turns to pain and localizes in the right lower quadrant, most frequently at a point two-thirds of the way between the navel and the very top of the right pelvic bone (anterior-superior iliac crest). This pain syndrome can be elicited from the patient by asking two questions: Where did you first start hurting? (belly button); Now where do you hurt? (right lower quadrant as described). Those answers mean appendicitis until it is ruled out. It is possible but unusual to have diarrhea with appendicitis. Diarrhea usually means that the patient does not have appendicitis. I find it helpful to ask the patient to walk and to watch how they do it. A person with appendicitis will walk with rather careful, short steps, bent slightly forward in pain. They certainly do not bounce off the examining table and walk down the hall to the bathroom. Anyone with springy steps most likely does not have appendicitis.

Sometimes even full laboratory and x-ray facilities can do no better in evaluating this diagnosis. As mentioned earlier, the ultimate answer will come from surgical exploration. If a surgeon has doubts, he might wait, with the patient safely in a hospital or at home under close supervision. But the patient with those symptoms should certainly be taken to a surgeon as soon as possible.

In the examination of the acute abdomen, several maneuvers can assess the seriousness of the situation. The first is the determination of guarding to palpation. If the patient has a rigid stomach to gentle pushing, this can mean that extreme tenderness and irritation of the peritoneum, or abdominal wall lining, exists. Use only gentle pushing. If there is an area of the abdomen where it does not hurt to push, apply pressure rather deeply. Suddenly take your hand away! If pain flares over the area of suspect tenderness, this is called "referred rebound tenderness" and it means that the irritation has reached an advanced stage. This person should be evacuated to surgical help at once.

What can you do if you are in the deep bush, say the Back River of Canada, without the faintest hope of evacuating the patient? Move the patient as little as possible. No further prodding of the abdomen should be done, as their only hope is that the appendix will form an abscess that will be walled-off by the bodily defense mechanisms. Give no food. Provide small amounts of water, Gatorade, and fruit drinks as tolerated. With advanced disease the intestines will stop working and the patient will vomit any excess. This will obviously cause a disturbance to the gut and possibly rupture the appendix or the abscess.

Treat for pain, nausea, and with antibiotics as indicated in the paragraph above on Gallbladder infection.

The abscess should form 24 to 72 hours following onset on the illness. Many surgeons would elect to open and drain this abscess as soon as the patient is brought to their control. Other surgeons would feel that it is best to leave the patient alone at this time and allow the abscess to continue the walling-off process. These surgeons feel that there is so much inflammation present, surgery only complicates the situation further. Within 2 to 3 weeks the patient may be able to move with minimal discomfort.

One form of therapy never to be employed when there is a suspicion of appendicitis is the use of a laxative. The action of the laxative may cause disruption of the appendix abscess with resultant generalized peritonitis (massive abdominal infection).

It is currently thought that there is no justification for the prophylactic removal of an appendix in an individual, unless he is planning to move to a very remote area without medical help for an extended period of time and it is known from x-ray that he has a fecalith (or stone) in the colon at the mouth of the appendix. Otherwise, the possible latter complications of surgical adhesions may well outweigh the "benefit" of such a procedure.

VOMITING

Nausea and vomiting are frequently caused by infections known as gastroenteritis. Many times these are viral so that antibiotics are of no value. These infections will usually resolve without treatment in 24 to 48 hours.

Fever seldom is high, but may briefly be high in some cases. Fever should not persist above 100° F (38° C) longer than 12 hours. Nausea may be treated with meclizine 25 mg every 8 hours from the Non-Rx Oral Medication Module or Atarax 25 mg every 6 hours from the Rx Oral/Topical Medication Module. If the Rx Injectable Medication Module is available, severe nausea and vomiting may be treated with Vistaril 25 to 50 mg every 6 hours given intramuscularly. Vomiting without diarrhea will not require the use of an antibiotic. If the vomiting is caused from severe illness, such as an ear infection, then use of antibiotic to treat the underlying cause is justified.

The nausea induced by high altitude is discussed on page 194.

Nausea associated with jaundice, see the sections on hepatitis, pages 168 to 169.

Nausea from ingestion of sea food, see paralytic shellfish poisoning; page 83, scromboid poisoning, page 84; and ciguatera poisoning, page 83.

See also, poisoning from plant or food ingestion, page 82; and poisoning from ingestion of petroleum products, page 83.

MOTION SICKNESS

To prevent and treat motion sickness, a very useful non-Rx drug is meclizine 25 mg, taken 1 hour prior to departure for all day protection. There is minimal drowsiness or other side effects with this medication. Transderm Scop, a patch containing scopalamine, has been developed for prevention of motion sickness, but this requires an Rx. Each patch may be worn behind the ear for 3 days. It is fairly expensive, but very worthwhile if you are prone to this malady. There tends to be a higher frequency of side effects in elderly people with this medication, consisting of visual problems, confusion, and loss of temperature regulation. A valuable drug to treat motion sickness is the Atarax 25 mg every 4 hours as needed from the Rx Oral/Topical Module, or the Vistaril 25 mg IM every 4 hours as needed from the Rx Injectable Module.

DIARRHEA

Diarrhea is the expulsion of watery stool. This malady is usually self limited, but can be a threat to life, depending upon its cause and extent. Diarrhea can be the result of bowel disorders such as diverticulitis or colitis, infectious diseases such as cholera, shigella, salmonella and many other creatures due to food or water contamination, and rarely with appendicitis and gallbladder disease. The serious infectious disease malaria can have diarrhea as a presenting complaint. Obviously diagnosing the cause of diarrhea can be of importance both in regard to the treatment and to estimate the danger to the patient.

DIVERTICULITIS is found in people over the age of 40 and is generally only a condition of the elderly. Diverticula are little pouches that form on the large intestine, or colon, from a weakness that develops over time in the muscles of its wall. These are of no trouble unless they become infected. Infection causes diarrhea, fever, and painful cramping. Treatment is with antibiotic such as the Floxin 400 mg every 12 hours.

COLITIS and other inflammations of the bowel cause repeated bouts of diarrhea. At times a fever may be present. These cases are chronic, and like diverticulitis, the diagnosis must be made with barium enema x-ray or colonoscopy. If in doubt, treat with Floxin 400 mg every 12 hours. These conditions require specific drugs for treatment, such as the steroids included with the Rx Oral/Topical and Injectable Modules, but unless the person has a prior history of these diseases, their use in the wilderness is inappropriate.

TRAVELER'S DIARRHEA is from infectious causes so that prevention seems an appropriate priority. Prevention is effected by staying alert. Water sources must be known pure or treated as indicated on pages 71-74. Tainted food should be avoided. Once freeze-dried food has been reconstituted, it should be stored as carefully as any fresh, unprocessed food. Be wary of fresh fruits and vegetables in developing countries. Peel all such items, or thoroughly rinse with purified water, or boil for 10 minutes minimum. Often, in countries lacking refrigeration, fruits and vegetables are "freshened" on the way to the market by sprinkling these items frequently with water from roadside drainage ditches. The use of human fertilizer makes this water very contaminated. This contamination is not eliminated by drying or wiping with a cloth. If the item being sold in the market is sold by weight, such as a melon, be careful! Some merchants inject roadside water into their product to increase its weight and value. Certain animal products are tainted in various parts of the world, particularly at specific times of the year. Know the flora and fauna which your expedition plans to utilize from local sources![6]

The definition of diarrhea is 2 to 3 times the number of bowel movements that are customary for an individual. These stools would be either soft, meaning that they will take the shape of a container, or watery, meaning that they can be poured. By definition at least one associated symptom of fever, chills, abdominal cramps, nausea, or vomiting must be present. This will generally mean 4 unformed stools in a day, or 3 unformed stools in an 8 hour period when accompanied by at least one other symptom listed above. The disease is generally self-limiting, lasting 2 to 3 days. As many as 75% of people will have abdominal pain and cramps, 50% will have nausea, and 25% will have vomiting and fever. An acute onset of watery diarrhea usually means that an enterotoxigenic E. coli is the cause, but shigellosis will also first present in this manner. Symptoms of bloody diarrhea or mucoid stools are frequently seen with invasive pathogens such as Shigella, Campylobacter, or Salmonella. The presence of chronic diarrhea with malabsorption and gas indicates possible Giardia. Rotovirus disease starts with vomiting in 80% of cases.

In a study of U.S. students in Mexico, the cause of diarrhea was found to be: enterotoxigenic E. coli 40%; enteroadherent E. coli 5%; Giardia lamblia and Entamoeba histolytica 2%; Rotovirus 10%; Aeromonas 1%; Shigella 15%; Salmonella 7%; Campylobacter 3%; and unknown 17%.

Various medications have been shown effective in preventing traveler's diarrhea, but a 1985 consensus of experts discouraged their use due to cost, exposing people to drug side effects, possible development of resistant germs due to antibiotic overuse, and the normally benign course of the disease. Pepto-Bismol 2 ounces (4 tablespoons) or 2 tablets taken 4 times daily can prevent this problem. Ugh! There is about 8 aspirin tablets worth of salicylate in that quantity of Pepto-Bismol. Prevention with antibiotic is effective, although not usually indicated. The choice of antibiotic for either prevention or treatment depends on where in the world you are traveling. For prevention in Mexico, doxycycline 100 mg taken once daily should suffice. Elsewhere in the world, Floxin 200 mg once daily (one- half of a 400 mg tablet) would be a better choice.

Treating diarrhea with Pepto-Bismol requires 2 tablespoons every 30 minutes for 8 doses. As most diarrhea in developing countries is from bacterial causes, the use of antibiotic can be very effective. A single dose of the antibiotic Floxin 400 mg can eliminate diarrhea instantly. Imodium, from the Non-Rx Oral Medical Module, may not be required if you have access to the Floxin. A dose of Imodium may be given simultaneously with the

Floxin. When using the Imodium, give 2 tablets at once, followed by 1 tablet after each loose stool with a maximum adult dose of 8 tablets per day. One tablet of the pain medication Lorcet 10/650 can also stop diarrhea, but it would be best to use the Imodium and/or Floxin if they are available.

ORAL FLUID REPLACEMENT THERAPY

Profound diarrhea from any source may cause severe dehydration and electrolyte imbalance. The non-vomiting patient must receive adequate fluid replacement, equaling his stool loss plus about 2 liters per day. An adult can replace these losses by drinking enough plain water. A child, or less healthy adult, will require electrolyte replacement in addition to the water. The Centers for Disease Control and Prevention recommends the following oral replacement cocktails to replace the losses of profound diarrhea:

Prepare two separate glasses of the following:

Glass 1)   Orange, apple or other fruit juice
(rich in potassium) ....8 ounces

Honey or corn syrup (glucose necessary for
absorption of essential salts)....................................$\frac{1}{2}$ tsp

Salt, table (rich in sodium and chloride)................1 pinch

Glass 2)   Water (carbonated or boiled) ....8 ounces

Soda, baking (sodium bicarbonate). ....$\frac{1}{4}$ tsp

Drink alternately from each glass. Supplement with carbonated beverages or water and tea made with boiled or carbonated water as desired. Avoid solid foods and milk until recovery.

Throughout the world UNICEF and WHO distribute an electrolyte replacement product called Oralyte. It must be reconstituted with adequately purified water. These packets can be hard to obtain and expensive in the United States, but an ideal source is from the voluntary health organization, IAMAT.[7]

If the patient is maintaining fluid balance with an effective oral rehydration therapy, such as the packets as indicated above, the additional glass of carbonated or bicarbonate water solution is not necessary. Other products which are considered safe for rehydration are Naturalyte®, Pedialyte®,

Infalyte®, and Pediatric®. Gatorade® is too high in carbohydrate and too low in sodium, potassium, and base to be considered a safe substitute, even with modification.

WATER DISINFECTION

Water can be purified adequately for drinking by mechanical, physical, and chemical means.

The clearest water possible should be chosen or attempts made to clarify the water prior to starting any disinfectant process. Water with high particulate count, with clay or organic debris, allows high bacterial counts and tends to be more heavily contaminated. In preparing potable, or drinkable, water we are attempting to lower the germ counts to the point that the body can defend itself against the remaining numbers. We are not trying to produce sterile water, that would generally be impractical.

The use of chlorine based systems has been effectively used by municipal water supply systems for years. There are two forms of chlorine readily available to the outdoors traveler. One is liquid chlorine laundry bleach and the other is Halazone® tablets. Laundry bleach that is 4 to 6 percent can make clear water safe to drink if 2 drops are added to 1 quart of water. This water must be mixed thoroughly and let stand for 30 minutes before drinking. This water should have a slight chlorine odor. If not, the original laundry bleach may have lost some of its strength and you should repeat the dose and let stand an additional 15 minutes prior to drinking.

Halazone® tablets from Abbott Laboratories are also effective. They are actually quite stable with a shelf life of 5 years, even when exposed occassionally to temperatures over 100° F (38° C). Recent articles in outdoor literature have stated that Halazone has a short shelf life and that it loses 75% of its activity when exposed to air for two days. Abbott Labs refutes this and has proven the efficacy of use for Halazone® sufficiently to receive FDA approval. A clue to their stability is that they turn yellow and have an objectionable odor when they decompose. Check for this before use. Five tablets should be added to a quart of clear water for adequate chlorination.

Chlorine based systems are very effective against virus and bacteria. They work best in neutral or slightly acid waters. As the active form of the chlorine, namely hypochlorous acid (HC10), readily reacts with nitrogen containing compounds such as ammonia, high levels of organic debris decrease its effectiveness. The amount of chlorine bleach or Halazone® added must be increased if the water is alkaline or contaminated with organic debris.

Iodine is a very effective agent against protozoan contamination such as Giardia lamblia and Entamoeba histolytica which tend to be resistant to chlorine. Further, iodine is not as reactive to ammonia or other organic debris by-products, thus working better in cloudy water. Tincture of iodine as found in the home medicine chest may be used as the source of the iodine. Using the commonly available 2% solution, 5 drops should be added to clear water or 10 drops to cloudy water, and the resultant mix should be allowed to stand 30 minutes prior to drinking.

The Armed Forces were responsible for developing a solid tablet that provided a source of iodine. Tetraglycine hydroperiodide is available as Globaline® or Potable Aqua®, or as Army surplus water purification tablets. An elemental iodine concentration of 3 to 5 ppm (parts per million) is necessary to kill amoeba and their cysts, algae, bacteria and their spores, and enterovirus. One tablet of Potable Aqua® will provide 8 ppm iodine concentration per quart. If the water is clear a ten minute wait is required; for cloudy water wait 20 minutes before consuming. At near freezing temperatures, wait a full 30 minutes before drinking.

Crystals of iodine can also be used to prepare a saturated iodine-water solution for use in disinfecting drinking water. Four to eight grams of USP grade iodine crystals can be placed in an one-ounce glass bottle. Water added to this bottle will dissolve an amount of iodine based upon its temperature. It is this saturated iodine-water solution which is then added to the quart of water. The amount added to procedure a final concentration of 4 ppm will vary according to temperature as indicated in the chart:

TEMPERATURE	VOLUME	CAPFULS
37° F (3° C)	20.0cc	8
68° F (20° C)	13.0cc	5+
77° F (25° C)	12.5cc	5
104° F (40° C)	10.0cc	4

*Assuming 2.5 cc capacity for a standard one-ounce glass bottle cap.

This water should be stored for 15 minutes before drinking. If the water is turbid, or otherwise contaminated, the amounts of saturated iodine solution indicated above should be double and the resultant water stored 20 minutes before using. This product is now commercially available as PolarPure® through many outdoor stores and catalog houses.

Mechanical filtration methods are also useful in preparing drinking water. They normally consist of a screen with sizes down to 6 microns in size which are useful in removing tapeworm eggs (25 microns) or Giardia lamblia (7 to 15 microns). These screens enclose an activated charcoal filter element which removes many disagreeable tastes. As most bacteria have a diameter smaller that 1 micron, bacteria and the even smaller viral species are not removed by filtration using these units. For water to be safe after using one of these devices it must be pre-treated with chlorine or iodine exactly as indicated above prior to passage through the device. While these filters remove clay and organic debris, they will plug easily if the water is very turbid. A concern with the charcoal filter usage is the possibility for them to become contaminated with bacteria when they are used the next time. Pre-treating the water helps prevent this. I have frequently used a charcoal filter system to insure safe, good tasting water after chemical treatment.

Another filtration method is perhaps one of the oldest, namely filtering through unglazed ceramic material. This was done in large crocks, a slow filtration method popular in tropical countries many years ago. A modern version of this old system is the development of a pressurized pump method. Made in Switzerland, the Katadyn Pocket Filter® has a ceramic core enclosed in a tough plastic housing, fitted with an aluminum pump. The built-in pump forces water through the ceramic filter at a rate of approximately ¾ths quart per minute. Turbid water will plug the filter, but a brush is provided to easily restore full flow rates. This filter has a .2 micron size, which eliminates all bacteria and larger pathogens. Pre-treating of the water is not required. There is evidence that viral particles are also killed by this unit as the ceramic material is silver impregnated which appears to denature viruses as they pass through the filter. This possibility is being evaluated by the FDA at this time. I have worked with many groups using this device and they have had many favorable comments. These units are not cheap, costing about $240.00 retail. They weigh 23 ounces.

Another method of water purification has been with us a long time, namely using our old friend, fire. Bringing water to a boil will effectively kill pathogens and make water safe to drink. One reads variously to boil water

5, 10, even 20 minutes. But simply bringing the water temperature to 150°
F (65.5° C) is adequate to kill the pathogens discussed above, and all others
besides. At high altitude the boiling point of water is reduced. For example,
at 25,000 feet the boiling point of water would be about 185° F (85° C).

This matter of the minimal length of time required to make water safe
to drink should be discussed further. Bringing water to a boil is the minimal safe time for preparation. At times fuel or water supply may be in short
supply and this minimal time must be used. It will never be necessary to
boil water longer than 5 minutes and the shortest time mentioned (just
bringing the water to a boil) will suffice for a safe drinking water. This water
will not be sterile, but it will be safe to drink.

Water may be obtained by squeezing any freshwater fish and from
some plants. Never drink urine or sea water, as the high solute content of
these liquids will only dehydrate you more and make the problem worse.
A solar still can be prepared for reprocessing urine, water from grass, etc.,
as indicated in Figure 7. In water poor areas, catching rain water may be
an essential part of routine survival. Be careful of melting ice: treat all ice
melt water as indicated above. There is a very strong chance of contamination of ice deposits.

SOLAR STILL

FIGURE 7. *Solar still condensing drinkable water from vegetation or contaminated sources. A solar still is very slow and produces minimal amounts
of water.*

HUMAN WASTE DISPOSAL

This is not only a matter of esthetics, but of primary preventative medicine.
Improper waste disposal on the wagon train heading west in 1840–1850's
caused vast epidemics of cholera in the trains that followed. Unbelievable
numbers of people were killed. Even in our wilderness areas, it is widely
acknowledged that the cleanest appearing streams are suspect of human

contamination. Most official campsites in the national park system have toilets constructed. These should always be used. Otherwise, human defecation should be buried at least 40 yards from a lake shore or stream run-off. Waste should be buried shallow, allowing rapid decomposition. Use biodegradable toilet paper, such as one would buy from a camping specialty store or for use in septic tanks. An inexpensive lightweight plastic trowel, ideal for digging a "cat hole," can be purchased at most specialty shops. For an expanded discussion of this topic, see the book, *The Basic Essentials of Minimizing Impact on the Wilderness*, by Michael Hodgson.[8]

CONSTIPATION

One of the popular wilderness medical texts has instructions on how to break up a fecal impaction digitally (i.e. using your finger to break up a hard stool stuck in the rectum). Don't let it get that far. In healthy young adults (especially teenagers), there may be a reluctance to defecate in the wilderness due to the unusual surrounding, lack of a toilet and perhaps swarms of insects or freezing cold. It is the group leader's responsibility to make sure that a trip member does not fecal hoard, i.e., fail to defecate in a reasonable length of time. Certainly one should be concerned after 3 days of no bowel movements.

To prevent this problem, I always include a stewed fruit at breakfast. The use of hot and cold in the morning will frequently wake up the "gastric-colic reflex" and get things moving perfectly well. If the five-day mark is approaching, especially if the patient—and they have become a patient at about this point—is obviously uncomfortable, it may become necessary to use a laxative. From the medical kit (non-RX Oral Medication Module) give 1 bisacodyl laxative tablet 5 mg at bedtime. If that fails, the next morning take 2 of the tablets. Under winter conditions, when getting up in sub-zero weather might prove abominable, or under heavy insect conditions, take these tablets in the morning, rather than at night, to preclude this massive inconvenience. Any laxative will cause abdominal cramping, depending upon how strong it is. Be expecting this.

HEMORRHOIDS

Also called "piles", this painful swelling is a cluster of varicose veins around the rectum. External hemorrhoids are small, rounded purplish masses which enlarge when straining at stool. Unless a clot forms in them, they are soft and non-tender. When clots form, they can become very painful, actually excruciating. Hemorrhoids are the most common cause of rectal bleeding, with the blood also appearing on the toilet tissue. The condition can be very painful for about five days, after which the clots start to absorb, the pain decreases and the mass regresses, leaving only small skin tags. Provide the patient with pain medication (non-Rx item) Percogesic® 2 tablets every 4 hours. The application of heat is helpful during the acute phase. Heat a cloth in water and apply for 15 minutes 4 times a day if possible. Avoid constipation, as mentioned in that section.

For local pain relief, apply dibucaine ointment every 4 hours from the non-Rx Topical Bandaging Module. If you are carrying the Rx Oral/Topical Module, also mix in equal portions of the Topicort .25% ointment to provide the anti-inflammation ability of a steroid.

HERNIA

The most common hernia in a male is the inguinal hernia, which is an out-pouching of the intestines through a weak area in the abdominal wall located above and on either side of the penis. A hernia can be produced while straining, either lifting, coughing, sneezing, etc. There will be a sharp pain at the location of the hernia and the patient will note a bulge. This bulge may disappear when he lies on his back and relaxes (i.e. the hernia has reduced). If the intestine in the hernia is squeezed by the abdominal wall to the point that the blood supply is cut off, the hernia is termed a "strangulated" hernia. This is a medical emergency, as the loop of gut in the hernia will die, turn gangrenous, and lead to a generalized peritonitis or abdominal infection (peritonitis is discussed under APPENDICITIS). This condition is much worse than appendicitis and death will result if not treated surgically.

The hernia that fails to reduce, or disappear when the victim relaxes in a recumbent position, is termed "incarcerated". While this may turn into an emergency, it is not one at that point. Most hernia caused by straining in adults will not strangulate. Further straining should be avoided. If lifting items is necessary, or while coughing, etc., the victim should protect himself from further tissue damage by pressing against the area with one hand, thus holding the hernia in reduction. It would be a rather awkward way to carry a canoe.

PAINFUL TESTICLE

If severe, provide support by having the victim lie on the insulated ground with a cloth draped over both thighs, forming a sling or cradle on which the painful scrotum may rest. If ambulatory, provide support to prevent movement of the scrotum. Cold packs would help initially and providing adequate pain and nausea medication as available is certainly appropriate. Antibiotic is not required unless a fever results.

Spontaneous pain in the scrotum, with enlargement of a testicle can be due to an infection of the testicle (orchitis) or more commonly to an infection of the sperm collecting system called the epididymis (epididymitis). Treatment of choice would be to provide antibiotic such as the doxycycline 100 mg 1 tablet twice daily, which is frequently employed for this problem. The Floxin 400 mg tablet twice daily is also frequently used. Pain medication should be provided as necessary.

The problem may not be due to an infection at all. It is possible for the testicle to become twisted, due to a slight congenital defect, with severe pain resulting. This "testicular torsion," as it is called, is a surgical emergency. It can be almost impossible to distinguish from orchitis. In a suspected case of torsion it is helpful to try to reduce the torsion. Since the testicle always seems to rotate "inward" one need only rotate the affected testicle "outward." This will often result in immediate relief of the pain. If one cannot achieve this, or if you are dealing with an orchitis, no harm is done; but if it is a torsion, you have saved the testicle and the trip. A person with severe testicular pain should be evacuated as soon as possible as infection or torsion can result in sterility of the involved side. An unreduced testicular torsion can become gangrenous with life threatening infection resulting.

BLADDER INFECTION

The hallmarks of bladder infection (cystitis) are the urge to urinate frequently, burning upon urination, small amounts of urine being voided with each passage, and discomfort in the suprapubic region—the lowest area of the abdomen. Frequently the victim has fever with its attendant chills and muscle ache. In fact, people can become quite ill with a generalized infection caused by numerous bacteria entering their blood stream. At times the urine becomes cloudy and even bloody. Cloudy urine without the above symptoms does NOT mean an infection is present and is frequently normal. The infection can extend to the kidney, at which time the patient also has considerable flank pain, centered at the bottom edge of the ribs along the lateral aspect of the back on the involved side (often both sides). While bladder infections are more common in women than men, they are not an uncommon problem in either sex. One suffering from recurrent infections should be thoroughly evaluated by a physician prior to an extended wilderness trip.

There have been many drugs developed for treating infections of the genito-urinary system. The antibiotics recommended for the Rx medical kits all work excellently here. Doxycycline 100 mg taken 1 tablet twice daily is very effective. Floxin 400 mg twice daily is ideal if the doxycycline seems ineffective. Generally 3 days is a sufficient length of time for treatment. Symptoms should disappear within 24 to 48 hours, or it may mean that the bacteria is resistant to the antibiotic and the other should be substituted.

For severe infections, with high fever which has not responded within 48 hours to oral antibiotic use, the injectable Rocephin 500 mg IM given twice daily in place of the oral antibiotic would be a superior choice.

Additional treatment should consist of drinking copious amounts of fluid, at least 8 quarts per day! At times this simple rinsing action may even cure a cystitis, but I wouldn't want to count on it. Use an antibiotic if it is available. Discomfort may be relieved by Percogesic from the non-Rx supplies, or one half a Lorcet 10/650 from the Rx Oral/Topical Module, but these are seldom required due to the rapid onset of relief following administration of the antibiotic. The Percogesic or the ibuprofen may be needed to treat the fever which accompanies such problems prior to the start of the antibiotic and during the early stages of therapy.

VENEREAL DISEASE

These infections are totally preventable by abstention, any other technique falls short of being foolproof. Most venereal infections cause symptoms in the male, but frequently do not in the female. Either may note increased discomfort with urination, the development of sores or unusual growths around the genitalia, and discharge from the portions of the anatomy used in sex (pharynx, penis, vagina, anus). Some venereal diseases can be very difficult to detect, such as syphilis, hepatitis B, and AIDS. Hepatitis B is rampant in many parts of the world with high carrier rates in local population groups. It can be prevented with a vaccine (see Appendix B). These are no vaccines against the other venereal diseases.

Gonorrhea is common and easy to detect in the male. The appearance of symptoms is from 2 to 8 days from time of contact and basically consists of a copious greenish-yellow discharge. The female will frequently not have symptoms. From the Rx kit provide doxycycline 100 mg twice daily for 15 days, to ensure adequate treatment of syphilis.

Syphilis has an incubation period of 2 to 6 weeks before the characteristic sore appears. The development of a painless ulcer (1.4 to 1/2 inch in size), generally with enlarged, non-tender lymph nodes in the region, is a hallmark of this disease. A painful ulcer formation is more characteristic of herpes simplex. The lesion may not appear in a syphilis victim, making the early detection of this disease very difficult. A second stage consisting of a generalized skin rash (generally which does not itch, does not produce blisters, and frequently appears on the soles of the feet and palms of the hands) appears about 6 weeks after the lesions mentioned above. The third phase of the disease may develop in several years, during which nearly any organ system in the body may be affected. The overall study of syphilis is so complicated that a great medical instructor once said, "To know syphilis is to know medicine." Treatment of primary stage syphilis is 15 days of antibiotic, as mentioned above.

Development of a clear, scanty discharge in the male may be due to chlamydia or other nonspecific urethral infections. Symptoms appear 7 to 28 days after contact. Women may have no symptoms. Treat with the doxycycline 100 mg twice daily for 15 days. Blood tests for syphilis should be performed before treatment and again in 3 months. Twenty percent of victims with nonspecific urethritis will have a relapse, therefore adequate medical follow-up after the trip is essential.

The herpes lesions can respond to Zovirax ointment applied frequently during the day until they disappear in 8 to 10 days. Zovirax capsules 200 mg taken 5 times daily for 10 days are effective during the acute phase.

Upon return home trip members who may have experienced a sexual disease should be seen by their physician for serology tests for syphilis, hepatitis B tests, chlamydia smears, gonorrheal cultures, herpes simplex titers, and possibly HIV studies for AIDS. Lesions or growths should be examined as possible molluscum contagiosum and venereal warts should be treated.

GYNECOLOGY

VAGINAL DISCHARGE AND ITCHING

This is frequently not a venereal disease. The most common cause is a fungal or monilia infection. This condition is more common in conditions of high humidity or with the wearing of tight clothes such as pants or panty hose.

A typical monilia infection has a copious white discharge with curds like cottage cheese. From the non-Rx Oral/Topical Module one can use the clotrimazole 1% cream. This formulation has been designed for foot and other skin fungal problems, but it will work vaginally as well.

A frothy greenish-yellow, irritating discharge may be due to Trichomonas infection. This can be spread by sexual encounters. The male infected with this organism generally has no symptoms, or a slight mucoid discharge early in the morning, noted before urinating. The treatment of choice is Flagyl (metronidazole) 250 mg capsule 3 times a day for 10 days, or 8 capsules given as one dose. This drug cannot be taken with alcohol. Sexual abstention is important until medication is finished and a cure is evident clinically. Flagyl was included in the Extended Module and is also the best drug available in the U.S. for the treatment of giardiasis.

A copious yellow-green discharge may be gonorrhea. Any irritating discharge that is not thick and white is best treated with antibiotic such as the doxycycline or Floxin. If sexual contact may have been the source of the problem, treat for 15 days to also kill any syphilis which may have been caught simultaneously. A douche of very dilute Hibiclens surgical scrub, or very dilute detergent solution, can be prepared and may be helpful. Very dilute is better than too strong. Frequent douching is not required, but this may be used daily for a while as required for comfort and hygiene.

MENSTRUAL PROBLEMS

Menstrual flow is best contained with a vaginally inserted pad, but be sure to have had experience with the chosen product prior to heading back-country. Most come with waxed disposable paper bags, but an inner bag of plastic should be carried if it will be necessary to pack out discarded pads. The Surgipad® from the Topical Bandaging Module will substitute as an outer sanitary napkin if none is available. Menstrual cramping can generally be controlled with ibuprofen 200 mg 1 or 2 tablets every 4 to 6 hours from the Non-Rx Oral Medication Module. While this medication is used as an anti-arthritic, its anti-prostaglandin activities make it an ideal medication for the treatment of menstrual pain. From the Rx Oral/Topical Module, if necessary, one could use Lorcet 10/650 1 tablet every 6 hours as required.

Menorrhagia, either excessive flow or long period of flowage, should be evaluated by a physician to determine if there is an underlying pathology that could or should be corrected. If the problem is simply one of hormone imbalance, this can frequently be corrected with the use of birth control pills with higher amounts of estrogen and lower progestogen content. Again, the physician should be consulted well in advance of the wilderness outing, so that these symptoms will have been brought under control by the time of the expedition.

SPONTANEOUS ABORTION

Bleeding during pregnancy is not unusual—twenty to thirty percent of women bleed or cramp during the first 20 weeks of their pregnancy. This is termed "threatened abortion" and is treated with bed rest as this usually decreases the bleeding and cramping. Ten to fifteen percent of pregnant women will go on to abort. As long as all products of the abortion pass, a "complete abortion," the bleeding and pain stop and the uterus shrinks back to its normal size.

An incomplete abortion, the expulsion of only a portion of the fetus or the rupture of the membranes only, will usually require a surgeon's care to perform a D&C, but not always. However, urgent evacuation is always mandatory. Watch for signs of sepsis, such as elevated temperature, and start antibiotic if possible. Give the Rocephin 1 gram IM, followed by 500 mg IM every 12 hours. The best oral antibiotic recommended for your kit would be the Floxin 400 mg every 12 hours. Give pain medication as necessary.

ECTOPIC PREGNANCY

In an ectopic pregnancy, spotting and cramping usually begin shortly after the first missed period. If a pregnancy test is positive and the woman has severe lower abdominal pain lasting more than 24 hours, you probably have a surgical emergency on your hands. A rupture of the uterine tube usually occurs at 6 to 8 weeks of pregnancy, while a rupture of the cornual pregnancy occurs at 12 to 16 weeks. The rupture causes massive blood loss with a rapid onset of shock and death when it occurs.

While other causes of spotting during pregnancy are possible, you are in no position to handle any of them in the wilderness. Evacuate this woman urgently.

If a woman is having spotting, lower abdominal pain, and the pregnancy test is negative, you are in no position to bet her life that she is not pregnant. Ectopic pregnancies have lower blood levels of β subunit HCG hormone. To detect and the test may, therefore, be falsely negative.

MISCELLANEOUS

DIABETES

Diabetic children or adults can have an active outdoor life, but first learning to control their diabetes is an essential process to be worked with their physician. The increased caloric requirement of wilderness exercise may range above an extra 2,000 calories per day, yet insulin dosage requirements may drop as much as 50%. The diabetic and trip partners must be able to identify the signs of low blood sugar (hypoglycemia)—staggering gait, slurred speech, moist skin, clumsy movements—and know the proper treatment, i.e. oral carbohydrates or sugar candies and, if the patient becomes unconscious, the use of injectable glucagon. Urine of diabetic outdoor travelers should be tested twice daily to confirm control of sugar. This testing should preclude a gradual accumulation of too much blood sugar, which can result in unconsciousness in its far advanced stage. This gradual accumulation would have resulted in massive sugar spill in the urine, and finally the spill of ketone bodies, providing the patient ample opportunity to increase insulin dosage to prevent hyperglycemia (too high a blood sugar level).

Storage of insulin in the wilderness, where it forgoes recommended refrigeration, is not a major problem so long as the supply is fresh and direct sunlight and excessive heat is avoided. Syringes, alcohol prep pads, Ketodiastix urine test strips, insulin and glucagon are light additions to the wilderness medical kit.

POISONING — INGESTION OF POISONOUS PLANTS OR FOOD

The Pittsburgh Poison Control Center manages the vast majority of their poison plant ingestion victims by treatment consisting of vomiting induced by syrup of ipecac. This technique provided totally adequate therapy. One-half oz of syrup of ipecac was given orally, followed with two 8 oz glasses of water to enhance vomiting. This technique provided superior emptying compared to gastric lavage (stomach pumping) and can even cause the expulsion of particles in the upper portion of the small intestine. If no vomiting occurs, repeat the dose of ½ oz of syrup of ipecac in 20 minutes. If all fails, induce vomiting by gagging the throat with a finger or spoon. This latter technique may well be the only method available while in the bush.

POISONING - INGESTION OF PETROLEUM PRODUCTS

The danger from accidentally drinking various petroleum products, say while siphoning from one container to another, is the possibility of accidentally inhaling or aspirating this liquid into the lungs. That will kill. The substances are not toxic enough in the GI tract to warrant the danger of inducing vomiting. Do not worry about swallowing several mouth fulls of any petroleum product. If the person vomits, there is nothing you can do about it, except position them so that there is less chance of aspiration into the lungs—sitting, bending forward is probably ideal. The more volatile the substance, the more the danger of aspiration. In other words, kerosene is less dangerous than Coleman fuel.

If organic phosphorous pesticides are dissolved in the fuel, you have a more complex problem. These substances are potentially toxic and must be removed. In the emergency room this would be accomplished by gastric lavage, or stomach pumping. In the bush, if you cannot evacuate the person within 12 hours, you will have to take a chance of inducing vomiting - with possible lethal aspiration—to eliminate the poison. Treat with ipecac or by inducing gagging as described under poison plant ingestion. After vomiting, administer a slurry of activated charcoal, if available. This helps bind unvomited toxins. Charcoal powder is available at pharmacies to which you add water to form the slurry. This substance and ipecac are common components of poison treatment kits.

CIGUATERA POISONING

This problem is caused by a toxin released by a small ocean organism called a dinoflagellate. As various species of fish eat this small plant they aquire the toxin. Larger fish that in turn prey upon these smaller fish acquire larger and larger amounts of the toxin and thus result in more severe cases of ciguatera toxin poisoning in humans. Over 400 species of fish from the tropical reefs of Florida, the West Indies, and the Pacific have been implicated. There is no change in flavor, texture, or color of the fish flesh and there is no way of detecting contamination. Worse yet, no method of preserving, cooking, or treating fish can destroy this toxin. One must rely on local knowledge to avoid potentially polluted species. As a rule of thumb, avoid the larger, more predatory, and older fish which are most likely to be contaminated.

Symptoms usually start with numbness and tingling of the lips and tongue, and then progress to dry mouth, abdominal cramping, vomiting and diarrhea that lasts 6 to 17 hours. Muscle and joint pain, muscle weakness, facial pain, and unusual sensory phenomena such as reversal of hot and cold sensations develop. Death may result from respiratory failure in severe cases. Treatment is supportive only as no specific antidote is available. See also the section on scromboid poisoning and paralytic shellfish poisoning.

SCROMBOID POISONING

The flesh of dark meat fish, such as tuna, mackerel, albacore, bonito, amberjack and mahi-mahi (dolphin) contain large amounts of histadine. Improper storage after catching these fish allows bacterial enzymatic changes of this meat, releasing large amounts of histamine and other toxic by-products which are not destroyed by cooking.

Symptoms of scromboid poisoning include flushing, dizziness, headache, burning of the mouth and throat, nausea, vomiting, and diarrhea. Severe poisoning can cause significant respiratory distress. Benadryl has been reported to cause an increase in symptoms at times which is surprising since it is an excellent antihistamine. Tagamet has been shown to block the effects of scromboid poisoning. While normally a prescription product used to control stomach acid formation, its mode of action is known as an H-2 histamine blocker. Other similar compounds in this class will have to be tested (Zantac, Pepcid, Axid), but if they are available they might be tried in an emergency.

PARALYTIC SHELLFISH POISONING

Mussels, clams, oysters, and scallops may ingest poisonous dinoflagellates known as the "red tide" during June to October along the New England and Pacific coasts. Numbness around the mouth may occur within 5 to 30 minutes after eating. Other symptoms are similar to ciguatera poisoning. These include gastrointestinal illness, loss of coordination, and paralysis progressing to complete respiratory paralysis with 12 hours in 8% of cases. No specific treatments or antidotes are available, but purging of stomach contents should be encouraged. Supportive medical care is available to alleviate symptoms. By this I mean intensive care unit supportive care with ventilator and IV medications to maintain blood pressure and general cardiovascular life support.

SOFT TISSUE CARE
AND TRAUMA MANAGEMENT

The first aid approach to a bleeding wound is to stop the bleeding, treat for shock, and transport the victim (with appropriate assessments) for definitive care. In remote areas, it will frequently be very appropriate for the party to provide its own definitive care.

Wound care, whether in the wilderness or not, can be broken into chronological phases. The first phase consists of SAVING THE VICTIM'S LIFE—by stopping the bleeding and treating for shock. Even if the victim is not bleeding, you will want to treat for shock. Shock has many medical definitions, but on the bottom line it amounts to an inadequate oxygenated blood supply getting to the brain. Lay the patient down, elevate feet above the head, and provide protection from the environment—from both the ground and the atmosphere. Grab anything which you can find for this at first—use jackets, pack frames, unrolled tents, whatever. Eventually you will be able to pitch a tent, put up a rain fly or sun shield, and prepare materials for further wound care. See also the discussion of shock on page 16.

Direct pressure is the best method of stopping bleeding—in fact pressure alone can stop bleeding from amputated limbs! When the accident first occurs, you may even need to use your bare hand to stem the flow of blood. Ideally, you will have something to protect you from direct contact with blood and to protect the wound from your dirty hand. The best item to carry would be a pair of vinyl gloves. They will stand long-term storage and heat/cold much better than latex gloves. At first you may have to grab a piece of cloth (bandanna, clothing article) or other barrier substance (plastic food wrapper). If direct pressure does not stop the bleeding, you may have to resort to the use of a tourniquet. Continue applying direct pressure while the tourniquet is on to facilitate the clotting process. Remove the tourniquet every 5 minutes, with continued direct pressure being applied, to see if adequate bleeding control can now be obtained with the direct pressure alone. Repeat this as often as necessary. Sometimes bleeding control with direct pressure may require hours of direct pressure, but this is unusual.

With the blood stopped, even with your hand, and the victim on the ground in the shock treatment position, the actual emergency is over. Their life is safe. And you have bought time to gather together various items you need to perform the definitive job of caring for this wound. You have also treated their fear and possible psychogenic shock. For obviously someone knows what to do: they have taken charge, they have stopped the bleeding, they are giving orders to gather materials together.

In the first aid management of this wound, the next step is simply bandaging and then transporting the victim to professional medical care. For those isolated in the wilderness who must provide long-term care for wounds, further management will go through several more phases: cleaning, closing, dressing, and treating complications of infection that could happen.

WOUND CLEANSING

Adequate cleansing is the most important aspect of wound management. Especially when in an isolated or survival situation, the prevention of infection is of critical importance and this can only be assured by aggressive cleansing techniques.

There is an adage in nature: "The solution to pollution is dilution." In wound care this means copious irrigation. The whole purpose of scrubbing a wound is to reduce the total number of potentially harmful bacteria. We won't get'em all out, but if the total number is sufficiently small, the body's own defense mechanisms can take over and finish the job for us.

To best provide water for irrigation, prepare sterile water. This can be done by boiling the water for 5 minutes. Lacking the ability to do this, try to use water that is fit for drinking (see page 71 for techniques of water purification). In a pinch, clean water from a stream or lake can be used as long as you are not downstream from a native village or a bloated, rotting moose.

Water irrigation is the mainstay of wound cleaning. The use of a bota bag or a squeezable plastic water cube with a small hole poked in it to provide a strong force of water is very helpful.

To provide adequate force to the irrigation stream, there are two items of potential importance. One is the bulb syringe (see Figure 8). The 1 oz model is adequate for most wilderness wounds. The other approach is to use a syringe (10 ml to 35 ml size) with a new device attached called a Zerowet Splashield® (see Figure 9). With either technique one can increase the velocity of the water to aid in dislodging debris and those all important germs.

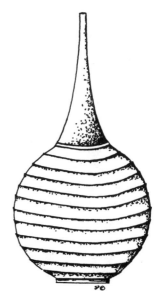

FIGURE 8. *The irrigating bulb syringe.*

FIGURE 9. *The Zerowet Spashield®—attached to a syringe.*

Adding surgical scrub solution to the irrigation water is not necessary to provide adequate wound cleansing. However, there are several products that can be particularly useful. The most effective is Hibiclens surgical scrub. Another is povidone-iodine diluted to a 1% solution (the stock solution is 10%). Another approach is to use very dilute soap solution. Err on the side of making the soap solution too weak, because strong soap solutions can damage healthy tissue. Make the solution weak enough that you could drink it without purging yourself.

There are many cleaning techniques and compounds that you should not use. Tincture of iodine, mercurochrome, or alcohol are very harsh—do not use. Hydrogen peroxide destroys good flesh as well as germs—do not use. Red hot branding irons and pouring gun powder into a wound and lighting it, while effective in killing germs and Rambo's favorite technique, also destroy good tissue and are similarly to be avoided.

Besides irrigation, there is a technique of cleaning used by physicians in the operating room called "debridement." This amounts to cutting away destroyed tissue. Of course, there is no way a person can do this in the bush—especially with inadequate lighting, equipment, and training. But we CAN safely approximate it by vigorously rubbing the area with a piece of sterile gauze or clean cloth. The rigorous scrubbing action will remove blood clots, torn bits of tissue, pieces of foreign bodies—all items which generally result in higher bacteria counts or foci for bacterial growth. This scrubbing process has to be accomplished quickly—it is painful and the victim will not tolerate it for long. Have everything ready: clean, dry dressing to apply afterward; the water supply; and instrument to spread the wound open (a splinter forcep is ideal); and sterile gauze to use for scrubbing the wound.

To sterilize cloth and any instruments, boil for 5 minutes, if necessary in the water you are preparing to use for irrigation.

While having adequate sterile dressings would be ideal, you may find yourself slicing and dicing your wool shirt or Polarguard jacket into bandaging material. A rough cloth works better at wound cleaning than a smooth cloth, such as cotton.

Once everything is ready, and assistance is at hand (perhaps someone to squirt the jet of water into the wound and another to assist shooing the black flies away or comforting the victim), go to it! If this job is performed well, the final outcome will be great. This part of wound care is far more important than wound closure technique. It will be messy. And it will hurt. But spread the wound apart, blast that water in there, scrub briskly with the gauze pad. This whole process will have to be completed in 20 to 30 seconds. In the operating room, or under local anesthesia in the emergency room, we might take 15 minutes or longer. You won't be able to take that much time, but you must be thorough and vigorous. When in doubt, you must do more—if the patient can tolerate it within reason.

Once completed with irrigation, the wound will be bleeding vigorously again; the blood clots having been knocked off during the cleansing process. Apply a sterile dressing and use direct pressure to again stop the bleeding. Use direct pressure as long as necessary to stop bleeding. Five to ten minutes usually suffice, but if an hour or more is required keep at it!

ANTIBIOTIC USE

It is always tempting to place a person on antibiotic after a laceration, but I would advise against doing this unless the wound was from an animal or human bite (page 104), the wound occurred in contaminated water, or there was an open fracture (page 122). Bacteria are jealous creatures and do not like to share their food source with other species. If an infection were to develop, it will generally be a pure culture, the other species originally contaminating the wound having been killed off by the body defense mechanisms and the winning bacterium. If the patient is on an antibiotic from the beginning, the winning bacterium is guaranteed to be resistant to your medication. If no antibiotic was used initially, then there is hope that the emergent bacterium will be sensitive to the antibiotic which you are about to employ.

If it is necessary to start a prophylactic antibiotic, from the Rx Oral/Topical Medication Module, use Floxin 400 mg twice daily. Use this for three days. In case of infection, see page 108.

WOUND CLOSURE TECHNIQUES

With direct pressure still applied, dry around the wound. We are ready to now enter the WOUND CLOSURE PHASE of wound care. Perhaps more worry and concern exists about this phase of wound care than the others, but it is really the easiest—and much less important than the first two phases just discussed.

TAPE CLOSURE TECHNIQUES

If the laceration can be held together with tape, by all means use tape as the definitive treatment. Butterfly bandages are universally available, and generally work very well. The commercial butterflies are superior to homemade in that they are packaged sterile with a no-stick center portion. They can be made in the field by cutting and folding the center edges in to cover the adhesive in the very center of short tape strips, thus avoiding adhesive contact with the wound. Of course such homemade strips will not be sterile, but in general they will be very adequate.

An improvement in the butterfly bandage was the Steri-Strip® by the 3-M Corp. I feel that today the best tape wound closure made is the Cover-Strip® by Beiersdorf, Inc. These strips drain fluid more readily and stick more firmly than Steri-Strips. Even better for amateur wound closers, they can be pulled off and reapplied when trying to correctly close the wound. Steri-Strips lose their stick once pulled up. If one end is pulled up to reposition it, then that strip is ruined.

In applying any type of tape closure, one technique is to pinch the wound together as the strips are being applied. That could take two people to accomplish. A simple one person method is to fasten a strip of tape to one edge of the wound and then fasten the next strip of tape to the other edge. Then approximate the wound edges by pulling on the tapes and fasten them down.

If taping will not hold the wound closed—and this may be the case when a stretch is placed frequently on the wound due to its location or to a gap due to missing tissue—then it will have to be stapled or sutured (stitched).

STAPLING

A new method of holding skin edges together is with the use of stainless steel staples. A special disposable device will contain a certain number of sterile staples which rapidly staple the wound edges while pinching the wound together. This obviously stings while being used, but the pain is brief and the wound is secure. A very useful such device is the Precise Five-Shot® by 3-M Corp, which obviously contains 5 staples. A special disposable staple remover is very handy for taking staples out virtually painlessly.

The skin stapler and staple remover are non-Rx. They come packaged in sterile, waterproof containers.

FIGURE 10. *The Precise Five-Shot-® Skin Stapler (left) and its companion staple extraction device (right).*

SUTURING (STITCHING)

Suture material is available in many forms and with many types of needles. For the expedition medical kit, I would recommend using 3-0 nylon suture with a curved pre-attached needle. This comes in a sterile packet ready for use. It will be necessary to use a needle holder to properly use this suture. The needle holder looks like a pair of scissors, but it has a flat surface with grooves that grab the needle and a lock device that holds the needle firmly. It is held as illustrated (see Figure 11) to steady the hand.

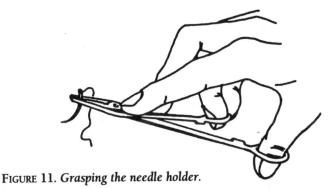

FIGURE 11. *Grasping the needle holder.*

Apply pressure in the direction of the needle, namely twist your wrist is such a manner that the needle will pass directly into the skin and cleanly penetrate, following through with the motion to allow the needle to curve through the subcutaneous tissue and sweep upward and through the skin on the other side of the wound. (Note illustration, Figure 12).

FIGURE 12. *Proper placement of suture, showing passage of the suture material at an equal depth on both sides of the cut.*

DEPTH OF SUTURES

Suture through the skin surface only and avoid important structures underneath. If tendon or nerve damage has occurred, irrigate the wound thoroughly as described above and repair the skin with either tape or sutures as necessary. The tendon, etc., can be repaired by a surgeon upon return to the outside—weeks later if necessary. If a delayed repair is necessary after a tendon laceration, the surgeon would probably wait a week to insure that a wound infection is not going to develop before attempting further surgery.

It is important to have the needle enter both sides of the wound at the same depth or the wound will not pull together evenly and there will be a pucker if the needle took a deep bite on one side and a shallow bite on the other (see Figure 13).

FIGURE 13. *Improper placement of suture, showing that different depths of penetration results in wound puckering.*

A square knot is tied with the use of the needle holder in a very easy manner. Loop the suture around the needle holder once, using the long end of the thread (see Figure 14A), then grasp the short end and pull the wound together (Figure 14B and C). Then loop the long end around the needle holder again the opposite way (Figure 14D). This will form a square knot. Repeat this process a third time in the original direction to insure a firm knot. Do not pull too tightly as this will pucker the skin, just an approximation is required. Frankly, a knot tied in any fashion will do perfectly well.

FIGURE 14.

B: Grasp end through loop.

D: Loop holder in reverse.

A: Loop holder.

C: Pull tight.

E: Grasp end through loop.

F: Pull tight.

SPACING OF STAPLES AND SUTURES (STITCHES)

These stitches should not be placed too closely together—usually, on the limbs and body 4 stitches per inch will suffice. On the face, however, use 6 per inch. Here it is best to use 5-0 nylon, as it will minimize scar formation from the needle and suture. I use a 6-0 suture on the face, but it is considerably more difficult to use than the 5-0. The use of these stitches can be augmented with tape strips or butterfly closures to help hold the wound together and to cut down on the number of stitches required. Once they are in, leave stitches in the limbs for 10 days, in the trunk and scalp for 7 days, and in the face for 4 days.

The number of sutures that are required can be minimized by placing Cover-Strips (or butterfly strips, etc) between the sutures. A wound that tends to break open due to tension, such as over the knee, can be stabilized by splinting the joint so that it cannot move while the wound is healing.

SHAVING THE WOUND AREA

It has been found that shaving an area increases the chance of wound infection. Scalp lacerations are hard to suture when unshaven due to the matting of hair with blood and accidental incorporation of hair into the wound. However, catching hair in the wound is not detrimental. Just pull it loose from the wound with a pair of forceps or tweezers when you are through suturing.

BLEEDING FROM SUTURE AND/OR STAPLE USE

Anywhere on the body you will note that entrance and exit points of the needle puncture will bleed quite freely. A little pressure always causes this bleeding to stop—it is not necessary to delay your sewing to even worry about it. Just complete your stitching of the wound, then apply pressure until the bleeding from the needle punctures stops, cleanse the skin when you are done to remove dried blood, and dress the wound.

SPECIAL CONSIDERATIONS

SCALP WOUNDS

Scalp wounds bleed excessively—be expecting this. Spurting blood vessels can be clamped with a hemostat and tied off with a piece of the 3-0 gut suture recommended for the Field Surgical Module. To tie, simply place a knot in the flesh to fall beneath the tip of the hemostat. Someone may have to remove the hemostat while you are cinching the first loop of the knot. Or you may simply suture the scalp wound closed and apply pressure between each suture to minimize intra-operative bleeding. Apply firm direct pressure after suturing to minimize hematoma—or blood pocket formation from bleeding within the wound.

I have read many times that a scalp laceration can be closed by tying the hair on either side into a knot, thus holding the wound together. I have sutured a lot of scalp lacerations and I doubt this technique would work very well. A scalp laceration bleeds profusely, blood is sticky and slippery at the same time, and the hair would have to be long enough and of the right texture—dreadlocks and the frizzies would not do.

EYEBROW AND LIP CLOSURE

If sewing an eyebrow or the vermillion border of the lip, approximate the edges first with a suture before sewing the ends or other portion of the laceration. Never shave an eyebrow. Use the 5-0 nylon suture on the face and remove these sutures in 4 days, replacing them with strips of tape at that time.

MOUTH/TONGUE LACERATIONS

When sewing the inside of the mouth, use the 3-0 gut suture. These sutures tend to unwind very easily, especially if the patient cannot resist touching them with his tongue. When making the knot, tie it over and over. As the mouth heals rapidly, if the sutures come out within a day, the laceration has generally stopped bleeding and may hold itself together without further help. These mouth sutures will generally dissolve on their own, but remaining ones can be removed within 4 days.

Lacerations on the tongue can almost always be left alone. The wound may appear ugly for a few days, but within a week or two there will be remarkable healing. Infections in the tongue or mouth from cuts are very rare. If the edge of a tongue is badly lacerated, so that the tongue is cut one-fourth the way across or more, then sewing the edge together is warranted. Use the 3-0 gut suture.

CONTROL OF PAIN

For anesthesia you will require a Rx to obtain injectable lidocaine 1% and a syringe with needle. Inject through the wound, just under the skin on both sides of the cut. Cleansing and suturing soon after a cut may help minimize the pain, due to tissue "shock" in the immediate post-trauma period. Ice applied to the wound area can help numb the pain, but local topical anesthetic agents like dibucaine are of no help in pain control. Two Percogesic or 1 Lorcet 10/650 given about 1 hour prior to surgery, may help minimize pain.

DRESSINGS

Most sutured lacerations will leak a little blood during the first 24 hours. The ideal covering would be the Nu-Gauze pads as mentioned on page 203. After the wound becomes dry, the Tegaderm dressing (page 202) will keep the sutures visible and the wound protected even if it must get submersed in water. Wounds that are leaking considerable serum and/or blood should be covered by Spenco 2nd Skin® and managed as discussed on page 203.

ABRASIONS

An abrasion is the loss of surface skin due to a scraping injury. The best treatment is cleansing with Hibiclens surgical scrub, application of triple antibiotic ointment, and the use of Spenco 2nd Skin® with Adhesive Knit Bandage—all components of the Non-Rx Topical Bandaging Module. This type of wound leaks profusely, but the above bandaging allows rapid healing, excellent protection, and considerable pain relief. Avoid the use of alcohol on these wounds as it tends to damage the tissue, to say nothing of causing excessive pain. Lacking first aid supplies, cleanse gently with mild detergent and protect from dirt, bugs, etc., the best that you can. Tetanus immunization should have been within 10 years.

A significant question on the mind of the victim and the medic is how aggressively should ground-in cinder and dirt be removed from a road rash. Having raced bicycles for several years on a cinder track (the Indiana University Little 500), I have had personal experience as a rashee. This, perhaps, clouds my perspective. Before I raced, these wounds were aggressively cleaned with a wire brush. During my racing year the approach changed to simply coating the wound with a layer of the antibiotic ointment and allowing the resultant scab formation to lift the cinders out of the wound when it fell off. A recent publication has shown that antibiotic salve, if applied within 3 hours of a surface wound, significantly decreases wound infection in animal studies.[9] I have not experienced problems with cinder tattoos or wound infections using gentle scrub with soft cloth, Hibiclens surgical scrub, removal of deeply imbedded debris carefully with tweezers, and a liberal coating of triple antibiotic ointment, reapplied daily or as necessary until the wound heals. I like to avoid a bandage, leaving the wound open to the air, or using the Spenco 2nd Skin®, when a covering is required, over the ointment.

PUNCTURE WOUND

Allow a puncture wound to bleed, thus hoping to effect an automatic irrigation of bacteria from the wound. Apply suction with the Extractor® (venom suction device) immediately and continue the vacuum for 20 to 30 minutes. Cleanse the wound area with surgical scrub or soapy water and apply triple antibiotic ointment to the surrounding skin surface. Do not tape shut, but rather start warm compress applications for 20 minutes, every 2 hours for the next 1 to 2 days, or until it is apparent that no subsurface infection has started. These soaks should be as warm as the patient can tolerate without danger of burning the skin. Larger pieces of cloth work best as compresses, such as undershirts, as they hold the heat longer. Infection can be prevented, or treated with antibiotics as described in the section on cellulitis above. Dressing should be with a clean cloth. If sterile items are in short supply they need not be used on this type of wound. Tetanus immunization should be current (see Appendix B).

SPLINTER REMOVAL

Prepare the wound with Hibiclens surgical scrub or other solution that does not discolor the skin. Minute splinters are hard enough to see. If the splinter is shallow, or the point buried, use a needle or #11 scalpel blade to tease the tissue over the splinter to remove this top layer. The splinter can then be pried out better.

It is best to be aggressive in removing this top layer and obtaining a substantial bite on the splinter with the splinter forceps (or tweezers), rather than nibbling off the end when making futile attempts to remove with inadequate exposure. When using the splinter forceps, grasp the instrument between the thumb and forefinger, resting the instrument on the middle finger and further resting the entire hand against the victim's skin, if necessary, to prevent tremor. Approach the splinter from the side, if exposed, grasping it as low as possible. Apply triple antibiotic afterwards.

Tetanus immunization should be current. If the wound was dirty, scrub afterwards with Hibiclens or soapy water. If deep, treat as indicated above under PUNCTURE WOUND with hot soaks and antibiotic as indicated.

FISHHOOK REMOVAL

The first aid approach to an impaled fishhook is to tape it in place and not try to remove it if there is any danger of causing damage to nearby or underlying structures or if the patient is uncooperative. Cut the fish line off the hook. Destroy triple hooks, but do not cut the hook close to the skin with your wire cutters. This makes subsequent manipulation by the surgeon more difficult.

If you will be longer than 2 days to reach help, it is important to remove any impaled object, to include a fishhook, as such objects are a high risk of causing an infection. And, since fishhooks are relatively easy to remove anyway, you may wish to do it yourself to prevent a long trip back to town and the doctor's waiting room.

There are three basic methods of removing a fishhook.

Push through, snip off method—While the technique seems straightforward, consider a few points: 1) Pushing the hook should not endanger underlying or adjacent structures. This limits the technique's usefulness, but it is still frequently an easy, quick method to employ. 2) Skin is not easy to push through. It is very elastic and will tent up over the barb as you try to push it through. Place side-cutting wire cutters, with jaws spread apart, over the point on the surface where you expect the hook point to punch through to hold the skin down while the barbed point punches its way to the surface. 3) This is a painful process and skin hurts when being poked from the bottom up, as much as from the top down. Once committed, get the push through portion of this project over with in a hurry. 4) This adds a second puncture wound to the victim's anatomy. Cleanse the skin at the anticipated penetration site before shoving the hook through using soap or a surgical scrub. 5) When snipping the protruding point off, cover the wound area with your free hand to protect you and others from the flying hook point. Otherwise you may need to refer to the section on "removing foreign bodies from the eye." The steps are simple: A) Push the hook through, B) snip it off, C) back the now barbless hook out, D) treat the puncture wounds. If you do not have wire cutters, you may still use this technique, but be able to crush the barb flat enough that you will be able to back the hook out.

The string jerk method—This is the most elegant of the methods. Fingers are loaded with fibrous tissue that tends to hinder a smooth hook removal. This technique works best in the back of the head, the shoulder, and most aspects of the torso, arms, and legs. It is highly useful and can be virtually painless, causing minimal trauma.

Important to the method is looping a line, such as the fish line, around the hook and insuring that this line is held flush against the skin. Pushing down on the eye portion of the hook (Figure 15 A) helps disengage the hook barb, so that the quick pull (Figure 15 B) will jerk the hook free with minimal trauma. Many times a victim has been quoted as asking "When are you going to pull it out?" after the job has been completed.

FIGURE 15A. *Press shank of hook against the skin surface.*

FIGURE 15B. *Vigorously jerk hook along the skin surface.*

The dissection method—But at times it just seems we are not to be so lucky and we have to resort to what will probably be a difficult experience for the victim and surgeon alike. This is the case of embedded triple hooks, a hook near the eye, or other situations when the above methods cannot be used. No person in his right mind would attempt this on his own if evacuation to a physician was at all possible. It is tedious, and without a local anesthetic such as injectable lidocaine, extremely painful.

The technique employs the use of either a #11 scalpel blade or an 18 gauge or larger bore hypodermic needle. Examine a hook similar to the one which is embedded in the victim to note the bend in the shank and the location of the barb. You will need to slide the blade along the hook shank, cutting the strands of connective tissue so that the hook can be backed out.

If using the needle, you will need to slide it along the hook and attempt to engage the barb, thus shielding connective tissue strands from the barb, allowing the hook to be similarly backed out. This is an elegant method and can result in minimal tissue damage, with only the entry hole left. But it can take time and without local anesthesia the victim would have to be stoic. If available, inject a little 1% lidocaine from the Rx Injectable Module. Practice using a piece of closed cell foam sleeping pad, rather than human skin, prior to your trip in the bush.

FRICTION BLISTERS

A relatively new and easily obtainable substance has revolutionized the prevention and care of friction blisters. The substance is Spenco 2nd Skin®, available at most athletic supply and drug stores. Made from an inert, breathable gel consisting of 4% polyethylene oxide and 96% water, it has the feel and consistency of, well most people would say snot. It comes in various sized sheets, sterile, and sealed in water-tight packages. It is very cool to the touch, in fact large sheets are sold to cover infants to reduce a fever. It has three valuable properties that make it so useful. One, it will remove all friction between two moving surfaces (hence its use in prevention) and two, it cleans and deodorizes wounds by absorbing blood, serum, or pus. Three, its cooling effect is very soothing, which aids in pain relief.

It comes between two sheets of cellophane. It must be held against the wound and for that purpose the same company produces an adhesive knit bandage. For prevention the 2nd Skin can be applied with the cellophane attached and secured with the knit bandaging. For treatment of a hot spot, remove the cellophane from one side and apply this gooey side against the wound, again securing it with the knit bandaging. If a friction blister has developed, it will have to be lanced. Cleanse with soap or surgical scrub and open along an edge with a #11 scalpel blade or equal. After expressing the fluid, apply a fully stripped piece of 2nd Skin. This is easiest done by removing the cellophane from one side, then apply it to the wound. Once it is adherent to the skin surface, remove the cellophane from the outside edge. Over this you will need to place the adhesive knit. The bandage must be kept moist with clean water. When used on an open or raw skin surface, the 2nd Skin should be replaced daily. Unless you have a friction blister and try using this stuff, you'll find it hard to believe how well it works!

Another product that provides pain relief and promotes rapid healing of friction blisters is the Unna boot included in the Orthopedic Module. This is the favorite item used by the British Army in treating this problem. Lance, collapse the blister, and wrap the zinc oxide impregnated Unna boot bandage around the foot or ankle with several wraps, cutting off the unneeded portion of this very long bandage and saving it for later use. I find it easiest to hold the Unna boot in place by covering it with a few wraps of an elastic bandage and then taping this securely.

BURNS

As soon as possible remove the source of the burn. Quick immersion into cool water will help eliminate additional heat from scalding water or burning fuels and clothing. Do not over cool the victim and cause hypothermia. If water is not available, suffocate the flames with clothing, sand, etc. Do not allow a victim to panic and run as this will fan the flames and increase the injury.

Treatment of burns depends upon the extent (percent of the body covered) and the severity (degree) of the injury. The percent of the body covered is estimated by referring to the Rule of Nines, as indicated in figure 16. An entire arm equals 9% of the body surface area, therefore the burn of just one side of the forearm would equal about 2%. The chest and back equal 18% and the abdomen and back equal 18%. The proportions are slightly different for small children, the head representing a larger percentage (18%) and the legs a smaller percentage (13.5%). Severity of burns is indicated by degree. First degree (superficial) will have redness and be dry and painful. Second degree (partial skin thickness) will be moist, painful, and have blister formation with reddened bases. Third degree (deep) involves the full thickness of the skin and extends into the subcutaneous tissue with char, loss of substance, or discoloration.

For purposes of field management, victims can be divided into three groups depending upon a combination of the extent and severity of the burn.

First degree burns, regardless of the extent, rarely require evacuation. The severe pain initially encountered in a 1st degree burn usually disappears within 24 hours. The patient's requirement for pain medication can range from ibuprofen 200 mg 4 tablets every 4 to 6 hours, Percogesic, 2 tablets every 3 to 4 hours, to Lorcet 10/650 1 tablet every 3-4 hours. After a few doses, further pain medication is generally not required. Surface dressings are not indicated, but soothing relief of small burns can be obtained by either applying a Spenco 2nd Skin® dressing or dibucaine 1% ointment.

FIGURE 16. *The "Rule of Nines" burn chart helps determine the percentage of a body covered by burns. Note the slight difference between an adult and a young child.*

Second degree burns covering less than 15% of the total body surface and 3rd degree burns covering less than 10% of the body surface area do not require rapid evacuation, but should receive professional care. Provide pain medication as above. Cleanse the area with either a surgical scrub or non-medicated soap. Do not attempt to remove debris that is stuck to the burn site. Gently pat dry. The general consensus is to remove skin from blisters that have ruptured or which are blood filled. I find it best to initially leave the skin covering on the blister, removing it after 3 days. People generally feel better when you open turgid blisters with a long cut using a #11 scalpel blade. Apply Spenco 2nd Skin® dressing and change twice daily. Second degree burns will slough the skin after 3 to 4 days. An unopened or covered blister surface will turn white in 3 days and frequently an ooze of pus may develop in the underlying blister fluid. If the underlying skin does not become red and swollen, this is a normal development. White moist dead skin should be cut away. If you have no ointment or dressings, leave a 2nd and 3rd degree burn alone. The surface of the blister, if it is drained, will dry out and slough off on its own. Either way, healing will take place in 2 weeks or less for a 2nd degree burn. A 3rd degree burn greater than 1/2 square inch will require a skin graft to heal. Red swollen skin under and around the burn site probably indicates an infection. If this develops, provide antibiotic from the Rx Oral/Topical Medication Module such as Cefzil 250 mg 2 capsules twice daily or from the Rx Injectable Module give Rocephin 500 mg intramuscular twice daily. Elevate the burned area to minimize the swelling.

A 3rd degree burn greater than 10% of the total body surface and 2nd degree burn greater than 15% of the total body surface area, any serious burn to the face and any 3rd degree burn of hands, feet, or genitals require urgent evacuation of the patient. Wound management is the least important part of the care of these patients. Burn wounds are sterile for the first 24 to 48 hours. Burn management is aimed at keeping the wound clean, reducing pain, and treating for shock.

An important aspect of treating for shock will be maintaining adequate fluid replacement. Generally patients with less than 20% of their body surface area burned can tolerate oral fluids very well. If they are not vomiting, those with between 20% and 30% of their body surface area involved can be resuscitated by drinking adequate fluids. This individual will be prone to go into shock. If the victim is vomiting, he will fall behind in fluid replacement.

The replacement fluid should initially consist of Gatorade diluted 1:1 with water or a mixture consisting of 1/3 teaspoon of salt and 1/3 teaspoon of baking soda in 1 quart of flavored, lightly sweetened water. Avoid the use of potassium rich solutions (orange juice, apple juice) as serum potassium can raise to high levels during the first 24 hours. During the second day the oral fluids should be diluted Gatorade and lightly sweetened, flavored water (such as Wylers or dilute Tang). Push as much fluid during these 2 days as the patient can tolerate without becoming nauseous. Attempt to keep urine flow 50 to 100 ml (1 2/3 ounce to 3 1/3 ounce) per hour. Nausea can be suppressed with adequate pain management and the use of Atarax 25 to 50 mg every 6 hours from the Rx Oral/Topical Medication Module or Vistaril

25 to 50 mg by intramuscular injection every 4 hours as needed from the Rx Injectable Module. Pain relief will require Nubain 10 to 20 mg intramuscular or the nasal inhaled Stadol® (see page 31) or the oral medications as tolerated. Patients who lapse into a coma during the first 48 hours will require intravenous fluids to save their life. Physicians equipped with IV fluids are aware of the massive doses that are required to succeed at this point.

Starting the third day the patient should be given a moderately high carbohydrate diet, rich in protein. Approximately 200 mg of Vitamin C and substantial Vitamin B complex should be started daily. This would equal about 4 each One-A-Day multiple vitamin (Miles) or equivalent. Continue to push fluids.

Spenco 2nd Skin® is the ideal burn dressing for these severe burns. It provides a breathable cover that is sterile and which will exclude bacteria from the environment. It is also easily removed with whirlpool or gentle cleansing. Otherwise apply a topical dressing such as triple antibiotic ointment. Occlusive dressings must not be used. The ointment may be placed on thick gauze dressings which are then held against the wound with a single layer of gauze roll dressing. The wound should be cleaned daily, removing obviously dead tissue. This can be done with gentle scraping using a sterile gauze and clean water with a little Hibiclens surgical scrub added, about one-half hour after proper pain medication has been provided. Lacking Hibiclens, use a very dilute soap solution. Elevate the burned area, if practical. Have the victim gently and regularly move the burned area as much as possible to minimize contraction of burn tissue across joints. This will only be a concern with long-term care lasting many weeks.

Avoid the use of oral or injectable antibiotics to prevent wound infection. If you suspect an infection has developed because the underlying tissue is becoming red and swollen, red streaks are traveling from the burn towards the heart, or the burn was grossly contaminated (such as from an explosion), use antibiotics as described above.

HUMAN BITES

Unless group discipline has really degenerated, human bites are due to accidents such as falling and puncturing flesh with teeth. Bites within the victim's own mouth seldom become infected and are discussed in the section on lacerations (see page 95). Human bites to any other location of the body have the highest infection rate of any wound. Scrub vigorously with Hibiclens surgical scrub, soapy water, or any other antiseptic that you can find. Pick out broken teeth or other debris. Use the Extractor® for 20 to 30 minutes, further use will not help. Coat the wound area with triple antibiotic ointment. Start the application of hot, wet compresses as described under puncture wounds. Start antibiotic with Rocephin 500 mg IM every 12 hours, or from the Rx Oral/Topical Module use Floxin 400 mg one every 12 hours or Cefzill 250 mg 2 tablets every 12 hours. Bite wounds to the hand are extremely serious and should be seen by a qualified hand surgeon as soon as possible.

ANIMAL BITES

Animal bites tend to be either tearing or crushing injuries. Animal bite lacerations must be vigorously cleaned, but hot soaks need not be started initially. Some authorities state that bite lacerations should not be taped or sutured closed due to an increased incidence of wound infection. This has not been my personal experience, nor that of many ER physicians with whom I have discussed this problem. After vigorous wound cleansing I would close gaping wounds as described under LACERATIONS. Puncture wounds should not be closed, only gaping wounds. Start antibiotic coverage immediately as described in the section on human bites. The massive lacerations from a large animal bite, such as bear or puma injuries, are another matter. The entire goal of treatment is to stop the bleeding, treat for shock, and evacuate. You may need to close these massive lacerations to help control bleeding.

If an infection seems to start, treat as indicated in the section on wound infection on page 108 by removing the closures and starting hot soaks and antibiotics.

Treat crush injuries with cold packs and compressive dressings.

Large lacerations can also be treated with compressive dressings. The ideal item would be a six-inch elastic bandage. Apply cold using chemical cold packs or the coldest water available, safely packaged in poly bottles or similar containers.

Refer to the section on rabies (page 172).

INGROWN NAIL

This painful infection along the edge of a nail can, at times, be relieved with warm soaks. There are several maneuvers that can hasten healing however. One technique is a taping procedure. A piece of strong tape (such as waterproof tape) is taped to the inflamed skin edge, next to—but not touching—

the nail. The tape is fastened tightly to this skin edge with gentle, but firm pressure. By running the tape under the toe, the skin edge can be tugged away from the painful nail and thus relieve the pressure.

Another method is to shave the top of the nail by scraping it with a sharp blade until it is thin enough that it buckles upwards. This "breaks the arch" of the nail and allows the ingrown edge to be forced out of the inflamed groove along the side. The above techniques should be implemented at the first sign of irritation rather than waiting for infection to develop, though even then they are effective. Provide antibiotics such as doxycycline 100 mg twice daily or Cefzil 250 mg twice daily.

PARONYCHIA

A paronychia is an infection of the nail base. This very painful condition should initially be treated with warm soaks, 15 minutes, every 2 hours, and the use of oral antibiotics such as the doxycycline 100 mg twice daily or the Cefzil 250 mg twice daily. Oral pain medication will also be necessary. If the lesion does not respond within 2 days, or if it seems to be getting dramatically worse, an aggressive incision with a #11 blade will be necessary (see Figure 17). This wound will bleed freely—allow it to do so. Change bandages as necessary and continue the soaks and medications as described under ABSCESS.

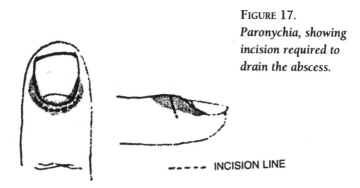

FIGURE 17.
Paronychia, showing incision required to drain the abscess.

----- INCISION LINE

FELON

A deep infection of a finger tip is called a felon. It results in a tense, tender finger pad. Soaking a felon prior to surgery, unlike other infections, does not help and only increases the pain. Treatment is effected by a very aggressive

FIGURE 18. *Felon, showing incision required to drain the abscess.*

incision, called a fish-mouth incision, made along the tip of the finger from one side to the other and extending deep to the bone! (See Figure 18).

An alternate incision is a through and through stab wound going under the finger bone, from one side to the other. A gauze or sterile plastic strip is then inserted through the wound to promote drainage of the pus from the felon.

The pain is severe and not helped by local injection of lidocaine. But relief is quick in coming as pressure from the pus build-up is then alleviated. Allow this wound to bleed freely. Soak in warm water for 15 minutes, every 2 hours until drainage ceases (about three days). Give pain medication about one hour prior to your surgical procedure, using the strongest that you have in your kit. Simultaneously start the victim on antibiotics such as the Cefzil 250 mg 2 tablets twice daily, the doxycycline 100 mg twice daily or the Rocephin 500 mg IM twice daily.

SUBUNGUAL HEMATOMA

This fancy term means blood under a fingernail or toenail. Generally caused by a blow to the digit involved, the accumulation of blood under a nail can be very painful. Relieve this pressure by twirling the sharp point of the #11 blade through the nail (using the lightest pressure possible) until a hole is produced and draining effected. Soak in cool water to promote continual drainage of this blood. Treatment for pain with Percogesic 1 or 2 tablets every 4 hours or Lorcet 10/650 one tablet every 4 to 6 hours, may also be necessary.

WOUND INFECTION AND INFLAMMATION

Lacerations which have been cleaned and either sutured, taped, or stapled together will generally become slightly inflamed. Inflammation is part of the healing process and does not indicate infection, yet the appearance is similar. It is a matter of degree. Inflammation has slight swelling and red color. The hallmarks of infection are: swelling, warmth to touch, reddish color, and pain. Pus oozing out of a wound is another clue. If the cut has a red swelling that extends beyond 1/4 inch from the wound edge, infection has probably started.

The method of treatment of wound infection is quite simple. Remove some of the tapes (sutures or staples) and allow the wound to open and drain. Apply warm, moist compresses for 15 to 20 minutes every 2 hours. This will promote drainage of the wound and increase the local circulation, thus bringing large numbers of friendly white blood cells and fibroblasts into the area. The fibroblast tries to wall off the infection and prevent further spread of the germs. Once an infection has obviously started, the use of an antibiotic will be helpful—but not always essential. From the Rx Oral/Topical Module use the Cefzil 250 mg 2 tablets twice daily, or the Floxin 400 mg 1 tablet twice daily. If the Rx Injectable Module is available, use the Rocephin 500 mg twice daily IM.

ABSCESS

An abscess (boil, furuncle) is a pocket of pus (white blood cells), germs, and red blood cells that have been contained by an envelope of scar tissue produced by fibroblasts. This protects the body from further spread of the germs. It is part of the body's strong natural defense against invasion by bacteria. Conversely, many antibiotics cannot penetrate into the abscess cavity very well. The cure of an abscess is surgical. They must be opened and drained. There are two basic ways in which this can happen. First, moist warm soaks will not only aid in abscess formation, but will also aid in bringing the infection to the surface and cause the infection to "ripen," even open and drain on its own. An abscess can be very painful and this opening period very prolonged. Once the abscess is on the surface it is generally better to open it using a technique called "incision and drainage" or I&D. The ideal instrument for an I&D is a #11 scalpel blade. This thin stab blade will penetrate the surface skin and open the cavity with minimal pressure on the wound. Abscesses are very painful, primarily because of the pressure within them. A person coming into a doctor's office with a painful abscess would expect to have it anesthetized before opening. Injections into these areas only add to the pain. The best anesthesia is to cool the wound area. In the field an ice cube or application of an instant cold pack will help provide some anesthesia. A person with a painful abscess will quite frankly let you try the knife as they can become desperate for pain relief. The relief that they get when the pressure is removed is immediate, even without cooling. Coat the skin surface around the abscess with triple antibiotic ointment from the non-Rx Topical Bandaging Module to protect the skin from the bacteria that are draining from the wound. Spread of infection from these bacteria is unlikely, however, unless the skin is abraded or otherwise broken.

CELLULITIS

Cellulitis is a very dangerous and rapidly progressive skin infection which results in red, painful swelling of the skin without pus or blister formation. The lesion spreads by the hour, with streaks of red progressing ahead of the swelling toward the heart. This represents the travel of infection along the lymphatic system and is frequently called "blood poisoning" in the vernacular. While lymphatic spread is not strictly blood poisoning, cellulitis does frequently lead to generalized blood poisoning (septicemia) and can cause the development of chills, fever and other symptoms of generalized profound infection such as lethargy and even shock. Very dangerous and virulent germs are responsible. Strong antibiotics are necessary. The application of local heat is very helpful. Old time remedies included the use of various "drawing salves," but nothing works better than local hot compresses. Local heat increases the circulation of blood into the infected area, bringing white cells which will kill the bacteria directly and which also produce antibodies to aid in killing the germs. The infection fighters, and the walling off process of the fibroblasts, will hopefully contain and destroy the infection. When this walling off process succeeds, then an abscess is formed (see previous section). If the Rx Injectable Module is available, give Rocephin 500 mg IM twice daily. Or, if only the Rx Oral/Topical Module is available, give Cefzil 250 mg 2 capsules twice daily or the Floxin 400 mg 1 capsule twice daily.

SKIN RASH

A rash is a frequent outdoor problem. At times a rash is associated with certain diseases and can help in the diagnosis. If the patient is feverish, or obviously ill, review the sections on Lyme disease, Rocky Mountain spotted fever, typhoid fever, syphilis, meningococcemia, strep throat, measles, and mononucleosis. Many infections which cause rash are viral and will not respond to antibiotic. But in the wilderness, with no professional medical help available, rash associated with symptoms of illness, particularly fever and aching, should be empirically treated with antibiotic such as the Cefzil 250 mg twice daily for at least 2 days beyond the defervescence (loss of fever). Some of the above infections require longer antibiotic treatment, so it should be continued as indicated if there is a probability that you are dealing with one of them.

Localized rashes without fever are usually due to superficial skin infections, fungal infections or allergic reactions. Itch can be treated with antihistamine or any pain medication. The Non-Rx Oral Medication Module has Benadryl 25 mg as an antihistamine. One capsule, two in severe cases, every 6 hours will help with itch from nearly any cause. As itch travels over the same nerves that carry the sensation of pain, any pain medication can also help with itch. Warm soaks generally make itch and rash worse and should be avoided, unless there is evidence of deep infection (see sections on CEL-LULITIS, ABSCESS above). It is hard to do better than Benadryl with regard to oral antihistamine effect, but it should be noted that Atarax (in the Rx Oral/Topical Module) and the same medication in injectable form, Vistaril (in the Rx Injectable Module), also have antihistamine action and can be used for itch. Also soothing to either a non-weeping lesion or a blistered and weeping lesion is the application of a piece of Spenco 2nd Skin® from the Topical Bandaging Module. Cool compresses will also sooth a rash.

If it is a moist, weeping lesion, wet soaks of dilute epsom salts, boric acid, or even table salt will help dry the lesion (this includes poison ivy, poison oak, and poison sumac). If it is a dry scaly rash, an ointment works the best, much better than a gel, lotion, or cream. Blistered rashes are treated best with creams, lotions, or gels. Specific types of rash require specific types of topical medications, however.

FUNGAL INFECTION

A fungal rash is commonly encountered in the groin, in the arm pit, in skin folds, on the scrotum, under a lady's breasts, and around the rectum. They can range from bright red to almost colorless, but are generally at least dull red and frequently have small satellite spots near the major portion of confluent rash. Fungal infections are very slow in spreading, with the lesions becoming larger over a period of weeks to months. Body ring worm is a circular rash with a less intense center area (Caution: see Lyme disease, page 169). Fungal rashes should be treated with a specific antifungal, such as the clotrimazole 1% cream from the Non-Rx Topical Bandaging Module. Either this product or miconazole 2% cream are the best antifungal medications that can be obtained without a prescription. Apply a thin coat twice daily. Good results should be obtained within 2 weeks for jock itch, but athlete's foot and body ring worm may take 4 weeks. If so, continue treatment until all evidence of rash is gone, then continue treatment once daily for an additional 3 weeks. If no improvement has been made, you may have the wrong diagnosis or a fungus that is refractory to your medication.

ALLERGIC DERMATITIS

The hallmark of an allergic dermatitis are vesicles, or small blisters, on red, swollen and very itchy skin. A line of these blisters clinches the diagnosis of allergic, or contact dermatitis. The most common reasons are poison ivy, poison sumac, and poison oak. Contact with caterpillars, centipedes, and many plants, even as innocent as various evergreen trees, can induce allergic or toxic skin reactions. A toxic reaction to a noxious substance, such as that from certain insects and plants, is treated the same as an allergic dermatitis. First aid treatment is a thorough cleansing with soap and water. Further treatment is with Benadryl 25 mg every 6 hours from the Non-Rx Oral Medication Module and twice daily applications of hydrocortisone cream 1% from the Topical Bandaging Unit. Weeping lesions can be treated with wet soaks as mentioned above. An occlusive plastic dressing will allow the rather weak 1% hydrocortisone to work much better.

The Rx Oral/Topical Medication Module has two very effective medications to treat this problem. Continue use of the Benadryl, but add Decadron 4 mg tablets, one daily for 5 to 7 days and apply the Topicort .25% Ointment in place of the hydrocortisone cream. A thin coat twice daily without an occlusive plastic dressing should work rapidly.

Stinging Nettle causes a severe irritation that can be instantly eliminated by the application of GI jungle juice, which is a 75% mixture of deet insect repellent and 25% isopropyl (rubbing) alcohol. I discovered this neat trick the hard way (accidentally) while camping in fields of the stuff along the Cape Fear River in North Carolina. Since mentioning this in the first edition of Wilderness Medicine in 1979, many others in contact with this plant have confirmed the treatment's instantaneous effectiveness.

BACTERIAL SKIN RASH

A common bacterial superficial skin infection causing a rash is impetigo. The normal appearance of this condition is reddish areas around pus filled blisters, which are frequently crusty and scabbed. The lesions spread rapidly over a period of days. The skin is generally not swollen underneath the lesions. Frequent places for it to start are around the nose and on the buttocks. It spreads rapidly from scratching and may soon appear anywhere on the body. Early lesions appear as small pimples, which form crusts within 12 to 24 hours. Lesions should be cleaned with surgical soap (or hydrogen peroxide) and then covered with an application of triple antibiotic ointment. Avoid placing bandages on these lesions as the germs can spread under the tape.

Bacterial skin infections generally must be treated with Rx antibiotics. From the Rx Oral Medication Module give Cefzil 250 mg twice daily. The Rx Injectable Medication Module contains Rocephin which would be ideal for this condition. Give 500 mg IM once daily. Treatment of cellulitis and abscess—forms of deep skin infections—are discussed on pages 109 and 108.

See page 55 for treatment of cold sores and lip or mouth lesions.

SEABATHER'S ERUPTION

The sudden onset of a very itchy rash associated with swimming in south Florida and the Caribbean is caused by larvae of the thimble jellyfish (*Linuche unguiculata*) or by the larvae of the sea anemone, *Edwardsella lineata*. The latter was shown to be responsible for thousands of cases on Long Island, New York. The rash appears as welts (urticaria) or as a fine red rash or pimply rash. It appears within 24 hours of exposure to ocean water, normally in areas covered by bathing suits. The tiny larvae are trapped next to the skin within the bathing suit and discharge nematocysts that cause the disease. Additional symptoms frequently associated with this rash include fever, chills, weakness, and headache, as the larvae penetrate the skin and cause illness. In south Florida the occurrence is from March to August, with a peak of outbreaks in May. In Long Island waters the outbreaks occur from mid-August until the end of the swimming season in early September. These outbreaks are episodic with very few cases some years and thousands of cases during peak years.

Treatment consists of topical corticosteroid (1% hydrocortisone cream from the Non-RX Topical Bandaging Module applied four times daily or .25% desoximetasone ointment from the Rx Oral/Topical Module applied twice daily) and antihistamine (diphenhydramine 25 mg from the Non-Rx Oral Medication Module 4 times a day). Swimmers should remove their bathing suits and shower as soon as possible after leaving the water. And swimming at a nude beach doesn't protect you from this just because you are not wearing a bathing suit.

ORTHOPEDIC INJURIES

Orthopedics includes the study of bone, joint and muscle function and disorders. The section establishes basic protocols for the assessment and care of orthopedic disorders. General concepts of care will be followed by a systematic assessment by anatomical region with suggested care plans.

The above table will refer you to general management principles and to diagnosis and treatment plans by anatomical region.

MUSCLE PAIN—NO ACUTE INJURY

Muscle aches can arise from chronic inflammation disorders such as lupus and fibromyalgia, but the discussion here will be limited to those conditions which might reasonably arise on a wilderness trek.

When associated with a fever consider an infectious basis for the pain. Without a reasonable method of diagnosis, it would be best to treat with both an antibiotic and appropriate pain medication. Even in North America, several serious conditions can present in this manner that require urgent treatment, such as Rocky Mountain Spotted Fever. Regardless of cause, it is appropriate to start ibuprofen 200 mg tablets, 2 to 4 tablets each dose, repeated every 6 hours, for fever and muscle ache.

While it's best to have a physician see the patient and to draw the appropriate lab tests before commencing antibiotics, if you are more than 2 days journey from treatment, start the doxycycline 100 mg twice daily or the Cefzil 250 mg twice daily. If you might be treating Lyme disease, this treatment will need to be continued for at least 2 weeks (see page 169).

Under conditions of heat stress, heavy exertion causing sweating, diarrhea, vomiting, or the use of diuretics causing increased urine output, a cause for muscle cramping is electrolyte abnormality. Appropriate fluid and electrolyte replacement is necessary as discussed on page 188.

Overuse syndromes cause pain in muscles that go beyond the mild ache you are accustomed to feeling after a workout at the gym. While it is possible to suddenly tear muscles with sudden movements, significant pain that starts gradually or after the exercise is over, can represent pain caused by a tendinitis, spasm caused by a pinched nerve, or significant inflammation in the muscle. The treatment for these conditions is the same as that employed for tendinitis as described in that section. Additionally, the use of a muscle relaxer is of benefit. From the Non-Rx Oral Medication Module take Percogesic 2 tablets every 6 hours or from the Rx Oral/Topical Module use Atarax 25 mg every 6 hours. These medications can be used in addition to the others prescribed for tendinitis unless the condition is relatively mild, then the use of Percogesic alone should suffice.

MUSCLE PAIN—ACUTE INJURY

Pain occurs immediately after a significant muscle injury, either a contusion or strain being the general cause. RICE is the acronym which applies here: Rest, Ice, Compress, Elevate. An elastic bandage, cold stream water, elevation of a limb, and rest may not all be possible, but they comprise the initial treatment. The application of cold is the most important, just do not cause freezing injury.

Contusions cause bleeding into the surrounding muscle tissue through the rupture of small blood vessels. RICE will minimize the bleeding and local swelling. Strains on muscles result in either microscopic muscle fiber tears or muscle mass tears. These are graded as Grade I (microscopic) to Grade IV (total tear of a muscle). Grades II and III are partial tears of a muscle mass. A total tear would require surgical repair. All will be treated alike in the wilderness setting. Initially use RICE, as indicated above. If significant swelling of the muscle occurs, consider that you are dealing with a Grade III or IV tear. Continue RICE for 2 days, otherwise use RICE for the first 24 hours.

The next step in treating significant muscle injury would be the application of local heat. In the case of minor injuries, apply the next day. For more serious injuries, delay the use of heat for 2 days. Continue the use of the compression dressing. Splint or sling as necessary for comfort. Decrease activity to a level where the pain is tolerable.

A full rupture of a muscle body will generally result in a bulging of the muscle mass and a loss of strength during the late recovery period. This may not be noticeable at first as the swelling would initially be deemed a result of local bleeding and the pain would restrict use. Once the pain is gone, continued swelling, especially after several weeks has passed, is probably due to a significant muscle tear or a ruptured tendon. This should be repaired when possible, but it is not a reason for an urgent evacuation.

JOINT PAIN—NO ACUTE INJURY

Pain in the joint without history of injury is generally due to an arthritis, bursitis, or tendinitis. Without a history of previous arthritis the latter two become more likely as the actual diagnosis, but the treatment is the same for all three. The most common reason for tendon or joint inflammation is not acute damage, but an overuse injury. Ancient French trappers frequently encountered an Achilles tendinitis while snowshoeing, which they aptly termed "mal de racquette." Persons hammering, chopping wood, or playing tennis are familiar with epicondylitis of the elbow (tennis elbow) which is a tendinitis of the elbow. Tendinitis can occur in the thumb, wrist, in fact any tendon in the body can become inflamed with over-use. Joints similarly become inflamed with repetitive activity or even unusual compression. Cave explorers and canoeists will, on occasion, encounter a patellar bursitis of the knees, and many people have formed bursitis flare-ups in a shoulder due to repeated employment of certain arm actions. Rafters, kayakers, and canoeists can develop tendinitis in the forearm due to the over-use of flexor tendons of the wrist.

Treatment of these conditions must include altering the activity which seems to have caused it. By changing a grip on an oar, using paddles with a different pitch to the blades, altering a movement to avoid generating additional pain, the victim can try to alleviate the discomfort and to reduce flaring it worse. Prior to an activity the application of heat to the sore area helps. Immediately after aggravating the condition, applying cold is a benefit. Within an hour return to a local heat application and continue this during the evenings. Applying a cream such as Mobisyl Analgesic Creme® with a dry heat might help a tendinitis as the active ingredient trolamine salicylate (10% concentration) penetrates the skin and provides local anti-inflammatory action. Sports creams that feel warm, such as Icy-Hot, etc., simply irritate the skin surface to cause an increased blood flow and thus provide warmth to the area. They do not have an anti-inflammatory effect and they do not provide any benefit over the application of heat.

If hot compresses seem to aggravate the pain, switch to a cold compress technique. Avoid making the movements which seem to cause the most pain for 5 to 7 days. Splinting may help during this period. Avoid non-use of the shoulder for longer than 2 weeks as it is prone to adhesion formation and loss of function can result.

The best medication for chronic joint pain is the ibuprofen from the Non-Rx Oral Medication Module due to its anti-inflammatory action. Four tablets every 6 hours will aid in the relief of joint and tendon pain. From the Rx Oral/Topical Medication Module one could use the Decadron 4 mg, given once daily for 7 days for joint inflammation. The Lorcet 10/650 may be necessary for pain relief, but it has no anti-inflammation activity like the ibuprofen.

JOINT PAIN—ACUTE INJURY

Immediately after a joint injury, the tendency is to want to evaluate the injury and thus determine how serious it is and to figure out how the injury may change the expedition plans. Frankly, making a precise diagnosis will probably not be possible and therefore our approach to the acute joint injury must look at methods of treatment and potential long-term care that takes this into account. The discussion in this book on orthopedic injuries considers the body by region and not by precise diagnosis of injury. Nevertheless, we must have some understanding of what might have happened, to make an accurate prognosis early in the event, and to minimize the damage and yet keep the victim as functional as possible. Unusual stress across a joint can result in damage to supporting ligaments. Ordinarily this is a temporary stretching damage, but in severe cases rupture of ligaments or even fracture of bones or tears of cartilage can result. These injuries are serious problems and may require surgical repair - this is best done immediately, but can safely be delayed 2 to 3 months. Fractures entering the joint space may result in long-term joint pain and subsequent arthritis. Cartilage tears do not heal themselves, unlike ligament, tendon, and bone damage. These frequently cause so much future pain and instability that surgical correction is required.

Proper care of joint injuries must be started immediately. Rest, Ice, Compression, and Elevation (RICE) forms the basis of good first aid management. Cold should be applied for the first 2 days, as continuously as possible. Afterward, applying heat for 20 minutes or longer, 4 times daily is helpful. Cold decreases the circulation, which lessens bleeding and swelling. Heat increases the circulation, which then aids the healing process. This technique applies to all injuries including muscle contusions and bruises.

Elevate the involved joint, if possible. Wrap with elastic bandage or cloth tape to immobilize the joint and provide moderate support once ambulation or use of the joint begins. Take care that the wrappings are not so tightly applied that they cut off the circulation. The Orthopedic Module of the medical kit has many items that provide safe, yet secure joint support. The Webril orthopedic padding, consisting of long strand non-woven cotton, wrapped around the joint and covered with an elastic bandage, is ideal if further swelling is expected. For a very secure wrapping, where no additional swelling is anticipated, use the Unna Boot bandage to provide a more rigid base and over-wrap with the elastic bandage.

Use crutches or other support to take enough weight off an injured ankle and knee to the point that increased pain is not experienced. The patient should not use an injured joint if use causes pain, as this indicates further strain on the already stressed ligaments or fracture. Conversely, if use of the injured part does not cause pain, additional damage is not being done even if there is considerable swelling. If the victim must walk on an injured ankle or knee, and doing so causes considerable pain, then support it the best way possible (wrapping, crutches, decreased carrying load, tight boot for ankle injury) and realize that further damage is being done, but that in your opinion the situation warrants such a sacrifice.

Under emergency movement conditions a boot should not be removed from an injured ankle as it may be impossible to replace it. However, one must avoid too much compression of the soft tissue swelling to prevent circulation impairment. Doing additional damage to the ankle and risking circulation damage to the rest of the foot is an important decision to make.

Pain medications may be given as needed, but elevation and decreased use will provide considerable pain relief. See also discussion of fractures below.

FRACTURES

A fracture is a medical term meaning a broken bone. It is not true that "if you can move the part it is not broken." Pain will prevent some movement, but this does not aid in the diagnosis between a fracture and a contusion. Fractures may be "simple," represented by a single crack in the bone, or "compound" with many cracks and pieces. There may be no way of telling which is present, or even if a fracture is there at all, without an x-ray. Deformity indicates either a fracture or contusion with soft tissue bleeding if located in the middle of a long bone area, or a possible dislocation or severe sprain with or without a fracture if located at a joint. The hallmark of a fracture is point tenderness or pain to touch over the site of the break. Swelling over the break site is further evidence of a fracture. Another way to deduce the presence of a fracture is to apply gentle torsion or compression to the bone in question with either technique causing increased pain at the fracture site.

Each fracture has several critical aspects in its management to consider: 1) Correct loss of circulation or nerve damage due to deformity of the fracture; 2) Prevent the induction of infection if the skin is broken at or near the fracture site; 3) Prevent further soft tissue damage; and 4) Obtain reasonable alignment of bone fragments so that adequate healing takes place. The non-skilled practitioner is limited to the first three management techniques.

The first aid approach to a fracture is to "splint them as they lie." This is not an appropriate response in remote areas. Straighten gross deformities of angulated fractures with gentle in-line traction (see Figure 19). Before straightening, check the pulses beyond the fracture site on both sides of the victim and check for any abnormality of sensation. After correcting the angulation the circulation should improve. As arteries and veins are hollow tubes, if they are forced to bend around a corner, their lumen will stretch and narrow, thus decreasing blood flow. When this bend is eliminated, the vessel will return to its normal size and blood flow will improve. As the person could be in shock, it might be difficult to feel the pulses on either side. A comparison is much more accurate than attempting to evaluate the circulation by examination of the injured side only.

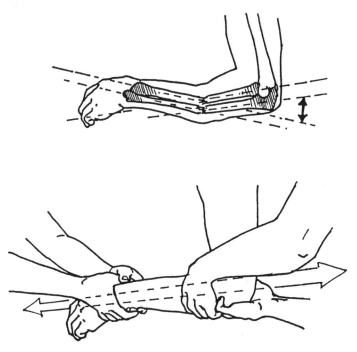

FIGURE 19. *Use traction-in-line to straighten grossly angulated fractures. This technique is not meant to perfectly align the bone ends and a hump deformity will still probably exist. This maneuver is only meant to eliminate gross deformity.*

Grossly angulated fractures also cause sharps ends of bone to project against the skin surface. Even with careful padding, jostling along during an evacuation may cause one of these bone spicules to penetrate the skin surface, causing an open fracture, increasing the chance of serious wound and bone infection.

The chance of causing harm while straightening an angulated fracture would be extremely low. It is possible for a blood vessel or nerve to become trapped within the fracture site, but gentle repositioning into slight deformity should correct this. Pad splints well to prevent skin damage. Pneumatic splints are available from many outfitters. Fracture splinting is generally well covered in first aid courses. Such a course should be taken before any major expedition into the bush. Improvisation is the name of the game in fracture immobilization and having an adequate first aid course provides one with information upon which to improvise. In general, splint fractures to immobilize the joint above and below the fracture site.

Any wound in the skin near a broken bone increases the chance of a bone infection. Follow the principles of thorough wound cleansing as indicated on page 87.

With proper splinting the pain involved with a fracture will decrease dramatically. Provide pain medication when possible. Pain control is discussed on page 30. The non-Rx Percogesic or Rx Atarax can be given to aid in muscle spasm control.

At times there will be uncertainty about whether a fracture exists. When in doubt, splint and treat for pain, avoiding the use of the involved part. Within a few days the pain will have diminished and the crisis may be over. If not, the suspicion of a fracture will loom even larger.

OPEN FRACTURE

Even a laceration or puncture wound near a broken bone is a cause for alarm. Such a wound can allow bacteria into the fracture site, causing a serious bone infection. This wound requires aggressive cleansing as indicated on page 87. The wound should not be closed as this increases the chance of infection. Wet dressings are best over an open wound. Soak the sterile dressing in sterile water, and cover with a clean dry dressing. Change this dressing twice daily.

If a piece of bone is protruding from the skin, the break is called an "open fracture." The first aid approach is to splint in position and cover with a sterile dressing. In a remote area this approach will not work. This wound will require aggressive irrigation with surgical scrub or soap as described on page 88.

The aggressiveness of this cleansing action should be done in such a manner as not to cause further damage, but the area must be free of foreign particulate matter and as antiseptic as possible. Cover the wound with triple antibiotic ointment. Protect with sterile gauze dressings, with enough pressure to control bleeding only. Straighten the gross angulation of the fracture with gentle in-line traction. This will cause the protruding bone to disappear under the skin surface, unless the fragment is loose from the main bone. Allow this wound to remain open and dress as indicated above.

In all cases of a laceration or puncture wound near a fracture, place the victim on oral antibiotics when available. From the Rx Oral/Topical Medication Module use the Cefzil 250 mg 2 tablets, twice daily. However, if the Rx Injectable Unit is carried, give the Rocephin 500 mg IM twice daily. Continue the medication until the patient is evacuated or the medication runs out.

DIAGNOSIS AND CARE PROTOCOLS

The diagnosis of these injuries will be difficult due to lack of experience or benefit of x-ray equipment. Uncertainties of diagnosis will exist and therefore a systematic approach to the evaluation and treatment of the injured patient will have to be developed that will handle most common injuries appropriately.

The orthopedic evaluation is made easier due to the fact that the human being has equal sides with which to make a comparison. Always take the clothing off the injured and the normal side and compare, weather permitting. Look for swelling or different configuration. When examining the injured side, touch lightly. A fracture or sprain is very tender and will not require hard poking to elicit obvious pain. Swelling is from local bleeding which a fracture will almost always cause. Several days after the injury a bruise may appear on the surface, or lower on the person as gravity will cause the spilled blood to migrate lower. Various muscle groups and local anatomy can also cause this blood to migrate to a place on the surface different from the injury site. This does not mean that the injury is spreading, but only represents the displacement of blood and part of the reabsorption process of healing. Do not be concerned about the appearance of bruising and its spread in the days after the injury.

HEAD[10]

The brain sits about one millimeter from inside your skull, comfortably in command of everything that goes on within you if the temperature, salt, water, blood sugar, and pressure stay balanced in your head. Head trauma ranges from simple scalp damage to severe brain damage. The severity is usually a result of the uncompromising structure of the skull (the cranium). If the brain starts to swell, it is squashed because there is no room up there for the swelling to take place.

For quick reference, head injuries can be divided into four categories:

1) NO LOSS OF CONSCIOUSNESS means only an extremely rare chance of serious problems, despite the fact that heavy bleeding and a huge goose-egg sized bump may accompany the injury. The brain has not been damaged.

2) MILD OR SHORT-TERM UNCONSCIOUSNESS tells that the victim's brain briefly contacted the inside of the cranium, and some transient loss of function occurred. There is usually nothing to worry about. Keep in mind the victim may not be aware they have been unconscious. Ask witnesses, if possible. Watch for the tell-tale signs of intracranial pressure (ICP), an announcement that the brain is being threatened:

   1. A headache that increases in intensity.

   2. Complaints of blurred vision or other disturbances.

   3. A level of consciousness progressing from disoriented to irritable to combative to coma.

   4. A heart rate slowing down and starting to bound.

   5. Noticeably irregular breathing, often progressing to deep and sighing breaths.

   6. Skin tending toward flush and warm, especially in the face.

   7. An increased blood pressure.

   8. Pupils becoming unequal in size with loss of normal reaction to light.

3) LONG TERM UNCONSCIOUSNESS is a serious warning that the ICP is on the rise. The problem may be a bruise to the brain, or a tear in the blood vessels of the meninges, or a laceration of the brain itself. The tough outer membrane (dura mater) may be clinging to the inside of the cranium, with blood collecting between the dura and the bone (an epidural hematoma). A subdural hematoma is blood pooling between the dura and the brain. The blood can gather over hours, or weeks, increasing pressure until death results.

4) OBVIOUS HEAD INJURIES include a depressed spot where the skull is fractured, visible fracture lines where a portion of the scalp has been torn away, black-and-blue around swollen eyes (Raccoon eyes), black-and-blue behind and below the ears (Battle's sign), and blood or clear 'cerebrospinal fluid (or both mixed) leaking from the nose or ears. Seizures are common.

To be safe, don't wait for the danger signals. Evacuate to professional medical attention anyone who has been forcibly knocked unconscious, even if they appear OK initially.

They can walk out if there are no obvious signs of injury. If there is a strong suspicion of injury, move them gently to prevent possible damage to their cervical spine, which is often at risk from a severe blow to the head. They need to have their entire spine immobilized. In the meantime, keep them lying down. If they must be left alone for any reason, roll them carefully onto their side to ensure an airway. Head injured people like to vomit, sometimes on a regular basis, and aspirated vomitus (vomit sucked into the lungs) usually causes death. Keep them lying down, on a slope if you can, with their head slightly uphill. You may be able to reduce the swelling rate of the brain with gravity's aid.

Once in a hospital, even the seriously head injured patient has a great chance of survival. Oxygen therapy, drug therapy, and surgical intervention are available. That's why they keep the patient awake, or arouse them regularly. If arousal is impossible, it is time for radical procedures. In a backcountry situation, let your patient fall asleep if they want to. In sleep the brain will have the best chance of controlling its own swelling. If your patient shows signs of improvement after 48 hours, their prognosis is very good.

While the use of pain and anti-nausea medication might alter the mental status and are avoided in urban first aid care, in a remote area during long-term care, providing these medications makes sense. It is best to use the mildest medication necessary for relief. Refer to the sections on pain management (page 30) and nausea management (page 66).

NECK

Examination of the neck is a critical task to help preserve the spinal cord from injury if the neck is unstable. Without moving the neck, gently palpate along the spinous processes to elicit point tenderness in the conscious patient. No point tenderness will generally mean no significant bone damage to the neck. In an unconscious patient with head trauma, treat as if the neck is fractured. Splint carefully for maximal immobilization. If the neck is at an odd angle, it should be straightened with gentle traction-in-line, by pulling steadily and slowly on the head along the line in which you find the neck. Move the neck to a neutral position with the spine in a line. This is a maneuver taught by wilderness first aid classes. Practice before attempting.

The patient should not be allowed to move, nor should they be lifted or transported without careful immobilization of the neck. The best technique of initial cervical immobilization is gentle but firm control by a person holding their head. Remind the victim to remain still. Eventually, this firm control can be replaced with a cervical collar or rolled ensolite pad or other soft material.

If no point tenderness is claimed by the conscious victim, but generalized pain and spasm of the neck muscles are present, the victim may be suffering a severe sprain. A neck brace made of a towel or other rolled cloth can help with the long-term treatment. Local warmth will help relax these muscles. Pain medication and muscle relaxants are useful in curing a neck sprain and spasm. It can take weeks for this injury to cease hurting.

SPINE

The neurological assessment of potential neck injury includes assessment of the entire spine. For a neurological check ask the patient if there is any numbness or tingling anywhere on their body. Check grip strength on both sides and the ability to wiggle toes and flex feet up and down. Check the entire spine by palpating along the spinous processes looking for any point tenderness. If the above examination is questionable, or even if the trauma seems severe, both neck and spinal immobilization are in order. Having a rescuer maintain firm hand control of the victim's neck will be necessary until the patient has been placed upon a suitable rigid stretcher. Rigid stretchers are very difficult to improvise; moving people upon them even more difficult. While *Medicine for the Backcountry* goes into great detail in describing this technique, these are skills that require practice (see page 229).

Ensure that the patient has been securely tied into the litter before you tie down the head. If the body were to shift with the head tied down, any damage present in the neck could increase.

In an urban environment, this is the end of the neck/spine story. The patient remains fastened rigidly to a stretcher until the Emergency Department physician has taken tests and made the determination that they can be removed. This may take several agonizing hours. I said agonizing, because even a normal person will hurt like crazy when attached to a rigid stretcher or back board. It's almost a self-fulfilling prophecy. If they didn't have back trouble when they were fastened down, they will when they are released. A recent study had 21 healthy volunteers (who had never experienced any back problems) placed in standard backboard immobilization for 30 minutes and found that 100% had pain during that period with 55% grading it moderate to severe, and 29% developed additional symptoms after release during the following 48 hours.[11]

Especially in a remote area setting, it will be important to reassess the spine to ensure that continued immobilization is really necessary. This is difficult if even normal people will develop back pain after a short time on the board. You will have to use common sense. Inability to move an extremity or loss of sensation, without an orthopedic injury in that limb, must cause a high suspicion of spinal cord injury. But if these signs and symptoms are not present and you become convinced that you are dealing with only a sore muscle problem in the back, not a broken or disrupted spine, then the spine may be cleared—a term meaning let them out of the rigid support. Continued partial support with a soft foam pad around the neck or even a back brace made of ensolite foam wrapped around them might make sense. Then again, it might not. It's a judgement call based upon severity of injury and resulting symptoms.

CLAVICLE (COLLARBONE)

Evaluate for pain to palpation along the collarbone or clavicle. Separations of the clavicle from the sternum (breastbone), fractures of the clavicle, and separations of the shoulder can all be treated similarly with a sling and swath.

To make a sling and swath, place the patient in a sling and then wrap the injured arm against the body with a wide cloth over the outside of the arm, running the cloth inside the other arm. A sling and swath will protect the injured shoulder and decrease pain in the recently fractured clavicle. This system can be duplicated by pinning the forearm to the front of a shirt. Use a sling without swath if there is a danger of the person slipping off a hill or falling into water.

The clavicle frequently fractures in the mid-portion. Proper reduction will occur if the shoulders are held back, like those of a Marine at attention. The common first aid "figure of eight" splint will maintain this position. Add a sling to improve stabilization and pain control. A swath further helps reduce movement and aid in reducing pain. Avoid allowing the person to assume a stoop shoulder position as this will allow too much override of the fractured parts.

A fracture of the clavicle at the end near the shoulder may be hard to hold in proper position. In children there is a sleeve of tissue at this location that aids in holding the proper alignment. In adults this tissue is missing and even surgical pinning may be required for optimal healing. However, even in the adult this fracture may be treated adequately usually with a sling and what other choice is there in the bush?

A fracture of the clavicle at the end near the breastbone (sternum) is best reduced and held in position with a figure of eight splint. In any clavicle fracture the use of a sling will aid greatly in decreasing pain. The sling can be eliminated in two weeks, but the figure of eight splint should be kept on for 3 to 4 weeks, or until there is no pain over the fracture site with free movement of the shoulder.

SHOULDER

Shoulder separations are classified as Grade I to Grade III depending upon the severity. Grade I is tenderness over the acromio-clavicular joint, the point at the very end of the clavicle, representing a strain of the ligaments but with no disruption or tear. A Grade II is a rupture of the two acromio-clavicular ligaments, which will result in a slight elevation of the clavicle. This elevation will be so slight that it probably cannot be seen, but there would be increased pain over the acromio-clavicular joint with weight bearing. Since increased pain is subjective, this diagnosis would be hard to make without a weight bearing x-ray. A Grade III strain is the disruption of both acromio-clavicular ligaments as well as the coraco-clavicular ligament. The latter case will allow obvious elevation of the clavicle at the acromio-clavicular joint as the entire suspension of the shoulder has been disrupted. There is no strong evidence that Grade III separations do better with surgery than without if they are willing to accept slight deformity at the end of the clavicle. Functionally they should do fine by treating with an arm sling for 3 to 6 weeks for comfort with mobilization of the shoulder as early as possible and return to activity.

Shoulder dislocations are separations of the humerus from the shoulder and are classified as either anterior or posterior. Anterior is by far the most common at a ratio of 10:1. Fractures of the head, or top part, of the humerus may be associated with dislocations. A reduction of the dislocation should be attempted as soon as possible. Muscle spasm and pain will continue to increase the longer the dislocation is allowed to remain untreated.

Anterior dislocations may be identified by comparison to the opposite side. The normal smooth rounded contour of the shoulder, which is convex on the lateral (outside) side, is lost. With anterior displacement the lateral contour is sharply rectangular and the anterior (or front) contour is unusually prominent. The arm is held away from the body and any attempted movement will cause considerable pain.

A numb area located just beneath the deltoid muscle means that the axillary nerve has been damaged. Numbness or tingling of the little finger could mean ulnar nerve damage, while decreased sensation to the thumb, index, and middle finger may mean the ulnar nerve is injured. These findings increase the urgency of attempting a reduction.

The best method of reducing the anterior dislocation of the shoulder is the Stimson Maneuver. While other methods exist, this technique puts less force on the shoulder which is particularly important in case fractures of the head of the humerus co-exist with the dislocation. The technique is illustrated in Figure 20. If the diagnosis is correct, there should be minimal pain using this technique. It usually takes at least 20 minutes for this method to work. The patient is aware of a sudden "clunk" as the shoulder reduces (relocates) properly. He has instant pain relief and is able to use the arm with minimal discomfort, if necessary, immediately. After reduction has been obtained, the arm is placed in a sling and a swath is wrapped around the arm and chest to hold the arm against the body for three weeks. Mobilization too soon after reduction will result in a weak, unstable shoulder. In a young person this sling and swath may be maintained for 4 weeks prior to range of motion exercise. Holding the position longer than 4 weeks will not reduce the chance of recurrent dislocation, while holding it there longer may result in a frozen shoulder.

FIGURE 20. *The Stimson Method of replacing a dislocated shoulder. Using a wide cloth, wrap the forearm several times. Attach this wrap to a bucket or bag filled with 10 to 15 pounds of rocks and allow gravity to do the rest.*

SCAPULA (SHOULDER BLADE)

Fractures of the scapula (shoulder blade) are generally due to major trauma and the patient may require treatment for multiple fractures of the ribs, punctured lung (pneumothorax) or heart contusion. A direct blow to the scapula may fracture it without these other injuries. Diagnosis is difficult without an x-ray, but suspicion may be high if there is point tenderness to palpation over the scapula, particularly several days after the accident. An indication of scapular fracture is Comolli's sign, which is a triangular swelling corresponding to the outline of the scapula. Treatment is with a sling and early mobilization to prevent stiffening of the shoulder.

UPPER ARM

The humerus is the upper bone of the arm. Fractures of the upper part (or head) of the humerus are most common in elderly people. Again, the shoulder will be very painful. The classification of these fractures is made with x-rays which would demonstrate that not only has a fracture occurred, but would indicate how many pieces and if angulation or displacement has transpired. Displacement or severe angulation frequently requires surgical repair, but often very conservative measures are followed by the orthopedic specialist. Without access to x-ray or an orthopedic specialist we will have to treat all injuries conservatively.

Fractures of the upper humerus are associated with swelling and eventual bruising of the shoulder and upper arm, with gravity slowly causing the swelling and bruising to appear lower and lower down the arm. Severe pain will prevent normal movement of the shoulder, but some movement is frequently possible. As fractures of the upper part of the humerus occur through bone that mends itself readily (cancellous bone), the final outcome is often more dependent upon limiting the length of time of immobilization and starting proper physical therapy than it is upon the number of pieces or the separation and angulation.

Conservative treatment will consist of a sling and swath. It is important in older individuals to mobilize the shoulder as soon as possible, otherwise adhesions form and a frozen shoulder results. An x-ray would help determine how much time should be allowed in the sling. This would range from only a few days to 4 or even 6 weeks for a fracture with marked displacement. If the patient is over 30 the best rule of thumb while treating without x-ray is to mobilize and start physical therapy at two weeks. A youngster can be left in the sling for 4 weeks. The therapy should consist of range of motion movements, such as circular elephant trunk motions while bending over, and raising the arm in front, to the side, and towards the rear. Effort should be made to move the shoulder as if the patient was wiping their bottom. All of this should be done by the patient without someone forcing their arm through these motions.

UPPER ARM FRACTURES (BELOW THE SHOULDER)

Fractures just beneath the head of the humerus—a region called "the neck"—will result in muscle spasm causing an overriding of the shafts of bone. This is prevented by applying a hanging cast. This amounts to a weighted cast applied to the forearm with a loop of cloth supporting much of the weight of the cast from around the victim's neck. Mobilization and physical therapy should be started in two weeks. It is not practical in a setting without x-ray to properly design and follow the results of a hanging cast. Pain and apparent fracture of the humerus at the shoulder will probably have to be treated with a sling and swath, with early mobilization as mentioned above.

Humeral shaft fractures take 2 to 4 months to heal. Located between the shoulder and the elbow, this is best splinted with a cast orthopedic surgeons call a "sugar tong" splint. It amounts to a U-shaped plaster extending from the arm pit around the elbow back up to the shoulder and molded to the arm after reduction and wrapped with an ace bandage. The Sam splint and elastic bandages provided with the Orthopedic Module can be used to construct a sugar tong splint.

Complete fractures of the shaft of the humerus will be exquisitely painful and unstable, even causing a crunching sound when the bone is gently stressed. Incomplete fractures will be very tender to touch. Several days after the injury, swelling and bruising will appear at the elbow and forearm. Humeral shaft fractures at a point one third of the way up from the elbow may cause damage to the radial nerve, thus causing numbness to the forearm and thumb and index finger. This numbness generally lasts from 3 to 6 months and will commonly resolve on its own. Developing a numbness is a serious consequence that reflects either a tear or compression on a nerve. This is an area where the development of such a numb feeling is less cause for panic.

ELBOW RELATED TRAUMA

Fractures of the humerus above the elbow are very treacherous as bone fragments may seriously injure the nerves or blood vessels at this location.

Fractures of the elbow itself are similarly dangerous due to the possible damage to nerve, blood vessel, or articular surfaces of the bones in this joint. The immense swelling associated with fractures or sprains at the elbow causes compression that frequently does more damage than sharp pieces of broken bone. Avoid splinting the elbow near a 90° angle. Allow the elbow to droop in the sling with a posterior padding. Never wrap the elbow joint at the front aspect - leave this area open to the air. It is compression in the front of the elbow joint, an area called the antecubital fossa, that frequently results in serious injury to the blood vessels and nerves. Surgical intervention with x-ray assistance is required to ensure normal elbow function under many circumstances with regard to elbow fractures. Allowing the injured elbow to freeze into a 120° position may be the only treatment you can offer under long-term survival conditions.

Dislocation of the elbow is most common in young adults. Fractures of the tip of the elbow frequently are involved, but generally do not cause future problems. Fractures of the condyles can cause severe problems as indicated above, primarily due to compression from associated bleeding on the neurovascular bundle. Reduction obviously should not be attempted if there is a chance of being treated properly by an orthopedic specialist with x-ray equipment. The appearance of the dislocated elbow would be obvi-

FIGURE 21. *The Stimson technique of reducing a hyperextension dislocation of the elbow. This dislocation results in forcing the ulna backwards so that the tip, the olecranon, become very prominent. Besides traction on the wrist, pushing on the olecranon aids in the reduction.*

ous when compared to that person's other elbow. Many people have a sharper appearance of the elbow tip than the average individual. However, swelling and a particularly prominent, hard point behind the elbow would indicate that a dislocation has transpired.

Pain medication should be given the victim to relax the muscles prior to attempting to reduce the dislocation. Figure 21 demonstrates the technique of reducing an elbow dislocation. You will note the similarity to the Stimson technique for reducing shoulder dislocations. With the patient on their stomache and the elbow bent over the edge of a table or ledge, either attach 10 pounds (4.5 kg) or manually apply downward traction on the wrist and guide the tip of the ulna (the olecranon) gently back into its original position.

The ideal position after reduction of the elbow is at 90° with a posterior plaster splint. A 90° position is potentially dangerous in that swelling may compromise the circulation. If the pulses at the wrist are decreased, then allow the elbow to droop as necessary to relieve this compression, possibly to a 120° position as described above. The reduction of a simple elbow dislocation is best maintained in the posterior splint for 3 weeks, then start range of motion exercises. Soaking the elbow in warm water about 15 minutes prior to starting the gentle exercise program is helpful. If unusual deformity has resulted, or if the elbow is frozen, this frozen position may have to be accepted under survival conditions, until definitive surgery can be accomplished later. Full and proper use of this elbow will probably never again be established, even after the delayed surgery.

FOREARM FRACTURES

Forearm fractures in children can generally be treated by reducing under x-ray and plaster casting, while in the adult they frequently are treated surgically. Both options are not available to the isolated wilderness inhabitant if evacuation is not possible. The position of splinting of forearm fractures differs depending upon the location along the two bones, due to different forces upon these bones from tendon and muscle attachments. This positioning can only be held properly with tight-fitting plaster splints. Bone alignment can only be followed through repeated x-rays. Therefore, it is obvious that a complete and unstable fracture of the forearm will very likely not heal properly when treated by crude techniques in a remote wilderness setting.

Most fractures of the forearm are not complete and unstable, however. They will heal nicely with protective splinting being the only required therapy. A stable crack can be suspected from swelling and point tenderness to gentle finger palpation by the examiner along the radius and ulna, the two forearm bones. Under this circumstance a splint must be manufactured that will provide stability so that this fracture can heal without danger of further trauma. The bone will weaken during the healing process and additional trauma may turn this non-displaced fracture into an angulated mess. Pad the splint well and provide a sling for at least three weeks. Keep splinted for a total of 6 weeks, longer if point tenderness is still present. If point tenderness disappears within a few days or at most 2 weeks, the injury was not a fracture, but simply a contusion, and the splint may be safely removed at that time.

Fractures associated with deformity in the forearm provide the physician with two challenges. First reducing the fracture and second maintaining its position with proper casting. Reduction of forearm fractures is generally done by traction, increasing the angulation to engage the fracture ends, then straightening the bones prior to casting. This is done with anesthesia. The survivalist had best splint deformed fractures of the forearm after straightening gross angulation with in-line traction. The splinted position will have to be maintained for 8 weeks or longer, depending upon the disappearance of local tenderness. A well-padded splint may generally be applied in a firm manner, immobilizing the elbow and wrist joints. Corrective surgery can be performed later. It is best avoiding a manipulation that will be extremely painful and which will be unstable anyway.

WRIST FRACTURES AND DISLOCATIONS

Wrist fractures and dislocations are common in young adults with the arm and hand extended in a fall. The three most common problems are fractures of the navicular (or scaphoid) bone, dislocation of the lunate, and perilunate dislocation. Navicular fractures frequently do not heal even with appropriate casting. Dislocations of the lunate or of the remaining carpals from the lunate would ideally be reduced, but without x-ray, experience, or at least local anesthesia this is not possible. Symptoms of lunate dislocation would be pain in the wrist and frequently numbness in the thumb, index, and middle fingers. There would be pain with any attempt to move the wrist. An abnormal nob on the palm side of the wrist at the crease, when compared to the other wrist, should be obvious to palpation. The numbness described indicates pressure on the median nerve from the dislocated navicular bone and an attempt at reduction should be made. With the wrist in extreme dorsiflexion, traction is applied while an attempt is made to push the lump back into position. The reduction often is accompanied with a pop which is quite obvious.

Perilunate dislocation will have similar symptoms and signs, with pain of attempted movement of the wrist and possible median nerve compression causing thumb, index finger, and middle finger numbness. The nob will not be present, but there will be a slight deformity of the back side of the wrist, sometimes called a modified silver fork deformity or hump at upper side (dorsum) of the wrist. The technique of reduction is similar, with traction being applied to the wrist and the rescuer's thumb placed firmly over the location of the lunate bone (just beyond the end of the ulna) to hold the lunate in position as the wrist is then gradually flexed to bring the rest of the carpal bones down into proper position with the lunate and the ends of the radius and ulna. There is generally no snap when this occurs. The numb feeling should wear off within the next hour if the pressure has been removed from the median nerve.

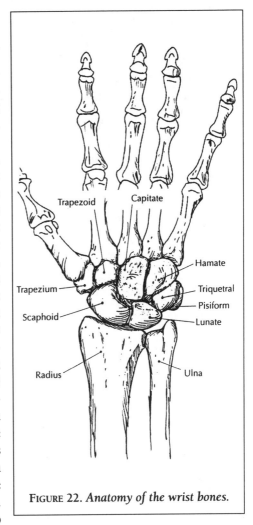

FIGURE 22. *Anatomy of the wrist bones.*

Navicular (scaphoid) fractures will have pain particularly on the thumb side of the wrist, and while the entire wrist will be sore to palpation, it will be particularly sore below the thumb at the wrist. This fracture seldom dislocates, but it is also prone to not healing, even after being placed in a tight plaster cast for several months.

After attempting to reduce a dislocation of the wrist and succeeding or

FIGURE 23.
Extreme dorsiflex-ion of the wrist. This is the position of the wrist used to aid in the reduction of the lunate bone dislocation.

not, or in treating the possible fracture of the navicular, it will be necessary to splint the wrist and thumb as immobile as possible. While it is not a rigid

dressing, a thick wrap using a two inch ace or Unna paste dressing applied in the manner called a thumb spica as illustrated (see Figure 24) can do fairly well. Under survival conditions fusion, arthritis, even loss of median nerve function, may have to be accepted. This is a terrible loss that proper orthopedic treatment can almost always avoid. The thumb spica wrap will be adequate for sprains of the wrist and thumb.

FIGURE 24.
The thumb spica wrap.

SPRAIN AND FRACTURES OF THE THUMB

Injuries causing severe pain and swelling of thumb may be sprains or fractures. A severe sprain will cause loss of strength of the thumb for many weeks, even months. Swelling can be substantial with either injury. The first aid management is splinting until treatment by a physician can be arranged. In an extended survival situation, reduce any obvious deformity and hold in position with a thumb spica wrap (see Figure 24). Severe sprains and all fractures will take 8 weeks to heal. There is risk of arthritis and loss of function depending upon the injury, patient's age, adequacy of reduction, and suitability of your splinting technique.

METACARPAL FRACTURES

A fracture of the 1st metacarpal will have to be treated with a thumb spica wrap that immobilizes the entire wrist. The 5th metacarpal is the most commonly broken bone in the hand. The name given to this fracture, a boxer's fracture, indicates its frequent method of origin. Perfect reduction of this fracture is not required, in fact up to 30 degrees of angulation can be accepted. Only five to ten degrees of angulation are acceptable in the 3rd and 4th metacarpals. Measuring the amount of angulation will be impossible without an x-ray, unless one is used to seeing these fractures frequently, then before and after x-rays become merely a legal maneuver and are not medically necessary. In the survival situation one may be able to tell if too much angulation has occurred by palpating the palm of the hand. If the nodular head of the metacarpal is felt where it joins the finger, there may be too much angulation. If too much angulation is allowed, the hand will be bothered throughout life with a lump in the palm of the hand, which makes holding tools and objects uncomfortable. Splinting should be maintained in a position of function for six weeks. Unacceptable angulation will have to be snapped back into place.

FRACTURES AND SPRAINS OF THE FINGERS

Gross deviations of fingers should be corrected and the finger splinted in the position of function. These deviations may be corrected by tugging and thus resetting the fracture or by placing a pencil or similar object between fingers and thus getting leverage to snap a deviated finger shaft back into place. Deviations at the joints probably represent dislocations and these may be easily reduced by the tugging technique generally. Swelling associated with "jammed" fingers can become permanent if use of the finger is allowed before adequate healing has taken place. After the acute injury, splinting in the position of function is always appropriate for at least three weeks, followed by buddy splinting to the adjacent finger for another two to three weeks. Fingers should not be splinted straight. Buddy splinting may be used initially if the victim must use the hand immediately, as in canoeing, etc.

Ruptured tendons can be repaired generally by splinting in a position of function with the exception of a rupture of the distal extensor tendon of a finger. This injury is rather common and can be caused by an object hitting the tip of the finger or catching the finger in something, a frequent occurrence being the snagging of a sheet while making a bed. While making beds may not be a problem of the wilderness, this illustrates how easy the injury may occur. Figure 25A illustrates the appearance of this injury, commonly called a mallet finger deformity. The splinting technique for this injury is not the position of function, but rather as illustrated in Figure 25B.

FIGURE 25A. *Mallet finger deformity from ruptured distal extensor tendon.*

FIGURE 25B. *Splint technique for the ruptured distal extensor tendon.*

HIP DISLOCATION AND FRACTURE

These injuries are very serious. Tremendous blood loss occurs internally. Fractures of the hip cause pain in the anterior medial aspect (front and side) of the thigh. Dislocations in younger people may be associated with fractures, in older people fractures are very common and are the probable cause of the deformity.

Posterior dislocation of the hip is more common in healthy young adults compared to central fracture-dislocations and anterior hip dislocations. All of these injuries are infrequent when compared, for instance, with dislocation of the shoulder. Posterior dislocations can cause injury to the sci-

FIGURE 26A.
Typical appearance of a fractured hip.

FIGURE 26B.
Typical appearance of a posterior hip dislocation.

FIGURE 26C.
Typical appearance of an anterior hip dislocation.

atic nerve, the main nerve of the leg. This can cause shooting pains down the back of the leg and/or numbness of the lower leg. It is most important that reduction of the dislocation not be delayed longer than 24 hours. Muscle relaxation and pain medication will be needed. To reduce, place the victim on their back with the knee and hip in a 90° position. The line of the femur should point vertically upwards. The thigh should be pulled steadily upwards while simultaneously rotating the femur externally (see Figure 27).

For evacuation purposes, pad well and buddy splint to the other leg. This victim is a litter case. Continued pressure on, or severe injury to, the sciatic nerve will cause muscle wasting and loss of sensation to practically the whole leg. This damage must be operatively repaired as soon as possible, or in the extreme case of survival without possible repair, bracing of the affected leg to allow mobility by the victim and care of numb skin areas to prevent sores and infection will be the only recourse.

Central fracture/dislocations result when the head of the femur is driven through the socket into the pelvis. As in all orthopedic injuries an x-ray is almost essential for the diagnosis. If the fragments can be replaced

FIGURE 27. *Reduction of the posterior hip disloca-tion, providing upward traction on the hip while flexed to 90° (panel A) and rotating externally (panel B)*

surgically, this is the treatment of choice. This injury can be left alone and still result in a stable and relatively painless joint. Light traction can be applied for comfort via adhesive tape applied to the lower leg. After three weeks ambulation with crutches with gradually increasing weight can be encouraged. Range of motion exercises of the hip should be started from the beginning to help mold the healing fragments into a relatively smoother joint surface. Sciatic nerve injury should not occur with this injury, but an arthritic joint will result.

Anterior dislocation results from forceful injuries as in airplane crashes and motorcycle accidents. The examination of the lower leg demonstrates considerable lateral rotation or outward tilting of the foot when the victim is laying on their back. Reduction is as described under posterior disloca-tion with traction on the flexed limb, but combined with medial rotation, or rotating the limb inward rather than outwardly.

FRACTURES OF THE FEMUR

Fractures of the femur can, of course, occur from the hip to the knee. They are classified and treated by the orthopedic specialist differently according to the locations of the break.

The first aid treatment consists of treating for shock and immobilizing, initially using a traction splint. Start by providing pain relief with gentle hands on in-line traction. Then rig a trucker's hitch or, weather permitting, tape directly to the skin to form the traction splint as illustrated.

Traction splinting is initially required as spasms from the powerful muscles in this region cause considerable overriding of bone fragments, increasing the extent of the injury. Traction also re-establishes the normal length and configuration of the musculature and tightens the membranes which surrounds the muscle (the fascia), which tends to decrease the bleeding that occurs with this injury. Additionally, the application of a proper traction splint can result in significant pain reduction. During prolonged transport, it is possible that the patient can be comfortably removed from the traction splint periodically. After several days, they may do quite well with buddy splinting to the other leg during litter transport. Prolonged use of the trucker's hitch traction splint system can lead to necrosis, or death, to the skin of the ankle due to the constant pressure. See Figures 28A and 28B.

DISLOCATED KNEE CAP (PATELLA)

The knee cap (patella) usually dislocates laterally, or to the outside of the knee. This dislocation results in a locking of the knee and the bump to one side makes the diagnosis obvious. Relocate the patella by flexing the hip and the knee. When straightening the knee the patella usually snaps back into place by itself. If not, just push it back into place while straightening the knee of the next try. Splint with a tube splint (ensolite foam), with the knee slightly flexed. This patient should be able to walk out.

KNEE SPRAINS/DISLOCATIONS/FRACTURES

The initial care of sprains, or acute joint injuries, is described on page 118. If the pain in the knee is severe, then several diagnoses are possible. There may be tears of ligaments, tendon, cartilage, and/or synovial membranes. There may be associated dislocations or fractures. All you really can assess is the amount of pain that the patient is having and you have to take his word for that. You can visually assess the amount of swelling or deformity and that might tell the tale, but the most important aspect of care will be the pain experience as the patient interprets it.

Have the patient lay as comfortably as possible. Rest, Ice, Compress, Elevate, (RICE) the knee. In case of significant pain and/or swelling, remove the boot (weather being feasible) and check the pulse on top of the foot (the dorsal pedal pulse) and question the victim about sensation in the feet. Check the dorsal pedal pulse on the opposite side for comparison. If the injury appears minor, this is not necessary.

Significant deformity means that a dislocation may have occurred. Serious disruption of the blood vessels and nerve damage can occur. Check

FIGURE 28A. *Application of webbing to form the Trucker's Hitch to prepare a traction splint in the field.*

FIGURE 28B. *The Trucker's Hitch attached to a ski pole padded with a shoe. This develops traction on the leg when pulled tight and tied off.*

the pulses and for sensation in the foot. If these are OK, splint the knee as it lies. If not, have a helper hold the lower thigh while you grip the ankle with one hand and the calf with the other. Use in-line traction while you gently flex the knee to see if you can reposition it better. If the pain is too great, you meet resistance, or you cannot do it, splint in the most comfortable position and evacuate as soon as possible.

Even without obvious deformity an immediate complaint, or continuing complaint, about significant pain means that you now have a litter case and you should make plans accordingly. If in two hours, the next morning, or two days later, the patient feels better and wishes to walk on it—great! Let them do it. You had best remove all weight from their shoulders and provide them a cane to use. Have them use the cane on the side opposite the injury. This places a more natural force vector on the injured joint. And continue the compressive dressing. After two days begin applying heat packs during rest stops and in the evening. The patient's perception of pain should be the key to managing these injuries in the bush, although this approach can be complicated by either a Macho or Wimp personality.

ANKLE SPRAINS/DISLOCATIONS/FRACTURES

Generally fractures of both sides of the ankle are associated with a dislocation. The severe pain associated with the fractures will be an early indication that this patient is a litter case. Splint the ankle with a single Sam splint or form a trough of ensolite foam and tape it on. The latter is not a walking splint, but if the pain is significant enough, the patient isn't walking anyway. A flail ankle, caused by complete disruption of the ankle ligaments, readily slops back into position and can be held in place with a trough splint of ensolite padding. Allow the patient to rest after the injury before attempting to walk on the ankle. If there is severe pain, it might be broken or badly sprained. Either way, if the pain is too severe, the patient ain't walking. At least not until it quiets down. As with the knee, if the pain diminishes enough that the victim can walk, allow them to do it without equipment and with a cane.

FOOT INJURIES

Stubbed toes can be buddy splinted to provide pain relief. If they have been stubbed to the extent that they deviate at a crazy angle sideways, they should be repositioned before buddy taping. Place a pencil (or a similar width object) on the side opposite the bend, and use it as a fulcrum to help snap the toe back into alignment. Blood under the toenail can be treated as described on page 107.

Severe pain in the arch of the foot or in the metatarsals can represent fractures or sprains. RICE as described above. Allowing a little time to lapse before use might result in decreasing pain in minor injuries, but it would take weeks for a fracture to decrease in severity. Decrease the patient's weight load and provide a cane. If the foot swells to the extent that the boot cannot be placed on the foot, consider cutting it along the sides and taping the boot on the foot. This provides support for the foot, ankle, and the patient's favorite outdoor retailer.

CHEST INJURIES

Broken ribs may develop after a blow to the chest. Even a severe cough or sneeze can also crack ribs! Broken ribs have point tenderness or exquisite pain with the lightest touch over the fracture site. The pain at this site will be reproduced by squeezing the rib cage in such a manner as to put a stress across the fracture site. Deep breathing will also produce pain at that location.

It is not necessary to strap or band the chest, except that such a band might prevent some rib movement and make the patient more comfortable. It is very important for the patient to be able to breath and have some cough reflex to aid in pulmonary hygiene - namely to prevent the accumulation of fluid in the lung which rapidly can lead to a pneumonia. Simply tying a large towel or undershirt around the victim's chest should suffice. A fractured rib will take six to eight weeks to heal. A similar pain may be initially present due to a tear of the intercostal muscles or separation of cartilage from the rib near the sternum or breast bone. These problems are treated as above. They heal much quicker, generally in three to five weeks.

If several adjacent ribs are broken in more than one location, a section of the chest wall is literally detached and held in place by the muscles and skin. This section of the chest wall can bulge out when the patient exhales instead of contracting as the chest normally would do. It can also move in when the rest of the chest expands during inhalation. This paradoxical motion of the chest is called a flail chest.

Treat all of the above conditions with pain medication as described on page 30. Avoid unnecessary movement. Have the patient hold their hand or a soft object against their chest when coughing to prevent rib movement and decrease the pain. Allow the patient to assume the most comfortable position which is usually sitting up. Treat with an antibiotic if fever starts, such as the Cefzil 250 mg twice daily.

Broken ribs usually heal well even though considerable movement seems to occur due to breathing or flailing of the chest. Fractured ribs are always so painful that the patients feel like they might puncture the lung at any minute. This does not usually happen, but if it does, there is a chance that air will leak into the chest cavity causing a pneumothorax. This can lead to significant respiratory distress to include cyanosis (blue discoloration of the skin due to inadequate oxygen in the blood). Crepitation can form in the skin. This is a crackling sensation that is very noticeable to the examiner when running the fingers over the skin in the upper part of the chest. It is not painful, but it indicates that a pneumothorax has occurred. A pneumothorax can resolve on its own or it can expand causing death. There is nothing which you can do for this unless you are trained in its management. Similarly, bleeding into the lung tissue can result in a hemothorax which can either resolve on its own or progress to death. Cyanosis with difficult breathing will also result due to this condition.

Section Five

BITES AND STINGS

For human bites, refer to page 104.

For animal bites, refer to page 105.

For aquatic bites/stings/cuts, refer to page 157.

For insect bites/stings, refer to page 145.

BEE STINGS

Stings from bees, wasps, yellow jackets, hornets (members of the Hymenoptera Family), and fire ants produce lesions that hurt instantly and the pain lingers. The danger comes from the fact that some persons are "hypersensitive" to the venom and can have an immediate anaphylactic shock which is life-threatening. Some non-stinging bites can also produce anaphylactic shock, namely the cone-nosed beetle (a member of the Reduviidae Family) located in California and throughout Central and South America.

The pain of the sting can be alleviated by almost anything applied to the skin surface. Best choices are cold compresses, dibucaine ointment from the Non-Rx Topical/Bandaging Module, and the use of oral pain medication such as Percogesic or stronger Rx medications as necessary. Delayed swelling can be prevented and/or treated with oral antihistamine such as Benadryl 25 mg taken 4 times daily from the Non-Rx Oral Medication Module. Sting relief is obtained with the application of the Sawyer Extractor (see page 149).

A generalized rash, asthmatic attack, or shock occurring within 2 hours of a sting indicates anaphylaxis, which requires special management.

ANAPHYLACTIC SHOCK

While most commonly due to insect stings, anaphylactic shock may be encountered as a serious allergic reaction to medications, shellfish and other foods, in fact anything to which one has become profoundly allergic. We are not born sensitive to these things, but become allergic with repeated exposures. Those developing anaphylaxis generally have warnings of their severe sensitivity in the form of welts (urticaria) forming all over their body immediately after exposure, the development of an asthmatic attack with respiratory wheezing, or the onset of symptoms of shock.

While these symptoms normally develop within 2 hours and certainly before 12 hours, this deadly form of shock can begin within seconds of exposure. It cannot be treated as indicated in the section on "normal" shock on page 16. The antidote for anaphylactic shock is a Rx drug called epinephrine (Adrenalin®). It is available for emergency use as a component of the Anakit® (use is described on page 215) or in a special automatic injectable syringe called the EpiPen®. I recommend the Anakit as it contains two injections of epinephrine, rather than one and the cost is about half that of the EpiPen. Normal dose use is .3 cc for an adult of the 1:1000 epinephrine solution given "subQ" (in the fatty layer beneath the skin). While it is not necessary to treat the itchy, generalized rash, the epinephrine should be given if the voice becomes husky (signifying swelling of the airway) and if wheezing or shock occurs. This injection may have to be repeated in 15 to 20 minutes if the symptoms return. The Anakit contains a chewable antihistamine which should also be taken immediately, but antihistamines are of no value in treating the shock or asthmatic component of anaphylaxis. Antihistamines can help prevent delayed allergic swelling and might be somewhat protective from irregular heart beats. If you have oral or injectable Decadron, give a 4 mg tablet or 4 mg injection for long-term protection which lasts during the next 12 hours.

A less expensive version of the Anakit is the AnaGuard®, which consists of only the syringe found in the Anakit, housed in a small protective plastic case. This would provide you with two adult injections of epinephrine at a retail cost in 1994 of less than $15.00. Two EpiPens retail for $80.00. The dose for persons under 12 years of age is one-half the adult dose which can be given by using the automatic injection EpiPen Jr. or by giving approximate amounts with the AnaKit/AnaGuard syringe.

Evacuate anyone experiencing anaphylactic reactions even though they have responded to the epinephrine. They are at risk of the condition returning and they should be monitored carefully over the next 24 hours. People can die of anaphylaxis very quickly, even in spite of receiving aggressive medical support in a hospital emergency department. Beyond 24 hours they are no longer at risk of an anaphylactic reaction. If the patient is still alive after that time, vital signs are stable, and there is no manifestation of anaphylaxis, the evacuation can be terminated.

SNAKE BITE

The main aspects of treating snake bites are to calm the victim, cause no additional harm, decide about evacuation urgency, and arrange for appropriate long-term wound care.

FIGURE 29. *The Anakit® and EpiPen® used to treat severe allergic reactions.*

How do you calm a person who has just be bitten by a snake? As with treating any disorder in this book, telling him to remain calm won't work. In a remote area when something terrible has happened, it's your actions which will provide comfort. Depending upon the individual, you may need to immediately treat for shock; you should certainly examine the wound. North American poisonous pit vipers will have left one or more fang marks. Some authorities feel that a proximal (on the leg or arm between the body and the bite site) constricting band should be applied—just do not make it too tight as you do not want to stop deep vein or artery blood flow. Do not pack the wound with ice. Do not place cuts in the wound or suck the wound with your mouth. Rubber suction cups do no good. The immediate application of the Sawyer Extractor (see page 149) is safe, effective, and very reassuring to the victim.

There is a golden hour and a half before the effects of North American pit viper venom causes significant generalized effects that might make the victim non-ambulatory. You might want to start walking the victim towards the road head to shorten the length of a litter evacuation. This walk out should be performed in a calm, but urgent manner.

Many bites by poisonous snakes inject no venom. The first symptom noted by many is a peculiar tingling in the mouth, often associated with a rubbery or metallic taste. This symptom may develop in minutes and long before any swelling occurs at the bite site. Envenomation may produce instant burning pain. Weakness, sweating, nausea and fainting may occur either with poisonous or nonpoisonous snake bites, simply due to the trauma of being bitten. In case of envenomation, within 1 hour there will generally be swelling, pain, tingling and/or numbness at the bite site. As several hours pass, ecchymosis (bruising) and discoloration of the skin begins and becomes progressively worse. Blisters may form which are sometimes filled with blood. Chills and fever may begin, followed by muscle tremor, decrease in blood pressure, headache, blurred vision and bulging eyes. The surface blood vessels may fill with blood clots (thrombose) and this can in turn lead to significant tissue damage after several days.

With regard to the visual identification of the most common poisonous snakes in North America, the pit vipers (Family Crotalidae which includes rattlesnakes, copperheads and water moccasins) take their names from the deep pit between the eye and nostril, which is a heat receptor organ. Most of them have a triangular head and they have a cat-like vertical elliptical pupil. Coral snakes (Micruruns fulvius, Family Elapidae), while not pit vipers, also have vertical elliptical pupils. Some nonpoisonous snakes do also. Color variations in coral snakes makes the old saying that if the "yellow is separated from the black, venom does it lack" (i.e. not a coral snake, but a king snake, etc.), a very treacherous method of identification. This is particularly true in Central and South America.

And now to look at the various considerations for handling both nonpoisonous and poisonous snakes.

TREATMENT OF SNAKE BITE

NONPOISONOUS SNAKE

Get away from the snake. Clean the bitten area with surgical scrub. Apply suction with the Extractor to promote evacuation of puncture debris. No constriction band should be used. Treat as under puncture wound on page 97. Tetanus immunization should be current.

PIT VIPER BITE

Not everyone bitten by a pit viper will have envenomation injury—fully 20% of rattlesnake and 30% of cottonmouth water moccasin and copperhead bites will not envenomate during their bite. 1) Immobilize the injured part at heart level or slightly above in a position of function. 2) Apply suction with the Extractor. Making incisions actually decreases the amount of venom that can be removed with this device. If applied within 3 minutes as much as 35% of the venom may be removed with the Extractor. After ½ hour, less than 3% more will be removed so further suction can be terminated. 3) Gently wash the wound with soap (or surgical scrub solution) and water. 4) Treat for shock (page 16), if necessary, and evacuate to professional medical help. DO NOT APPLY COLD—this is associated with increased tissue damage. Steroids should not be given routinely when caring for poisonous snake bites.

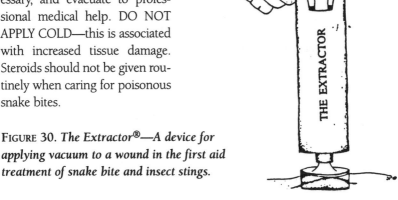

FIGURE 30. *The Extractor®—A device for applying vacuum to a wound in the first aid treatment of snake bite and insect stings.*

ANTIVENIN

Wyeth produces a polyvalent Crotalidae antivenin, which comes in a freeze-dried form. This may be stored for fairly long periods at room temperature. Each kit has a small bottle of horse serum to skin test the potential recipient, as the antivenin is made from horse serum. Many people are highly sensitive to the horse serum and it is possible that for these people this antivenin preparation may be more lethal than the snake bite. The test dose of the horse serum must be kept refrigerated. It would seem that members of an expedition heading into poisonous snake-infested areas could ideally be tested for sensitivity to the horse serum prior to departure. This would then allow the administration to be made without waiting 15 minutes for a skin test. It would also allow the non-refrigerated transport of the antivenin sets. However, this is dangerous as even skin testing can cause sensitization to develop in the individual and may result in anaphylactic shock upon giving the supposedly safe antivenin. I mention this idea simply to warn against trying it. However, a physician can order a special test called a Radio-allergosorbent Test (RAST) that can determine probable sensitivity to horse serum without exposure to it. The use of the antivenin, and the quantities to be given are described in the brochure that comes with each ampule. Generally, the minimal amount needed by an adult would be 3 amps; for a child 5 amps. For a swollen hand 5 to 8 amps IV would be given initially, with another 8 ready to go if the swelling progresses. Severe envenomation may require over 38 amps! This antivenin is only available by prescription and the current wholesale drug cost is $200.00. Approximately 7 to 10 days later, recipients of so much horse serum will develop a delayed reaction called "serum sickness." This will generally have to be treated with antihistamines (such as Benadryl) and steroids (such as Decadron). The use of the Wyeth Antivenin is not practical in the field and I would not suggest carrying it, even on snake gathering expeditions. Large doses given even several days after the attack can reduce apparent tissue damage considerably.

CORAL SNAKE BITE

The envenomation by this snake is via a slow chewing process, so that rapid withdrawal from the attack may have resulted in no uptake of venom by the victim. For treatment: 1) Treat for shock as necessary; 2) Wash the bitten area promptly; 3) Apply suction with the Extractor; 4) Avoid incisions; 5) Apply an elastic bandage with a firm wrap from the body towards the bite site, leaving the bite exposed if you have an Extractor for further treatment, covered if you do not; 6) Treat as a puncture wound and note tetanus precautions (pages 97 and 222).

Since the Coral Snake is an elapid, like the cobra, signs and symptoms of envenomation take time to develop and deterioration then proceeds so rapidly that the antidote may be of no avail. Many experts feel the antidote should be given immediately after skin testing in all cases. Most authorities feel 2 units of the Wyeth Micrurus fulvius antivenin should be given IV immediately. Some would use 10 amps of the antivenin. Note the discussion below under cobra bites.

COBRA, RUSSELL'S VIPER, GREEN MAMBA, KRAIT BITES

Most areas of the world have a local source of antivenin for the species of snakes that are of concern in that locale. In Africa many of the antivenins come from the Union of South Africa, but trade is greatly restricted to many other African countries. The use of a class of compounds called anti-cholinesterases can be lifesaving when dealing with neurotoxic envenomation, particularly if the antivenin is not available. A suggested protocol is the administration of .6 mg of atropine IV (.05 mg/kg for children) to control intestinal cramping followed by 10 mg of Tensilon (.25 mg/kg for children). If there is improvement, further control of symptoms can be obtained by titration of a dose of neostigmine .025 mg/kg/hr by IV injection or continuous infusion. I have provided this recent information for the benefit of a physician member of a party that might be at risk, although the medications are not included in the recommended Rx Injectable Unit.

SPIDER BITES

Generally spiders will make a solitary bite, rather than several. If a person awakens with multiple bites, he has collided with some other arthropod most likely. While only some spiders are considered poisonous, all spiders have venom that will cause local tissue inflammation and even slight necrosis or destruction. Most spiders are unable to bite well enough to inject the venom.

BLACK WIDOW

Latrodectus mactans

The black widow is generally a glossy black with a red hourglass mark on the abdomen. Sometimes the hourglass mark is merely a red dot or the two parts of the hourglass do not connect. At times the coat is not shiny and it may contain white. The bite may only be a pin-prick, but generally a dull cramping pain begins within one quarter of an hour and this may spread gradually until it involves the entire body. The muscles may go into spasms and the abdomen becomes board-like. Extreme restlessness is typical. The pain can be excruciating. Nausea, vomiting, swelling of eyelids, weakness, anxiety (naturally), pain on breathing may all develop. A healthy adult can usually survive, with the pain abating in several hours and the remaining symptoms disappearing in several days.

An ice cube or cold pack on the bite, if available, may reduce local pain. A specific antidote is available (*L. mactans* antivenin from Merck & Company) which should be given (after skin testing) to persons under 16 and over 65, heart or kidney patients, or those with very severe symptoms. The dose is one vial diluted in 15 to 50 ml of saline and given by IV over ten minutes. A specific treatment for relieving muscle spasm is methocarbamol (Robaxin) 100 mg given as a bolus into an IV line at 1 ml/min. After the initial bolus, a constant infusion of 200 mg/hr IV or 500 mg by mouth every 6 hours can be used. This medication has not been included in the Wilderness Medical Kit, but adequate pain relief can be sought by using the Percogesic from the Non-Rx Oral Medication Module, or the Lorcet 10/650 and Atarax from the Rx Oral/Topical Unit.

BROWN RECLUSE
Loxosceles reclusa and related species

A brown coat with a black violin marking on the cephalothorax or top part of the spider identifies this spider. The initial bite is mild and may be overlooked at the time. In an hour or two, a slight redness may appear; by several hours a small bleb appears at the bite site. At times the wound begins to appear as a bull's eye with several rings of red and blanched circles around the bite. The bleb ruptures, forming a crust, which then sloughs off; a large necrotic ulcer forms which gradually enlarges. Over the first 36 hours, vomiting, fever, skin rash and joint pain may develop, and hemolysis of the blood may be massive.

Apply ice to the wound as soon as possible. An antivenin has been developed from rabbits and is being used experimentally. Dapsone 100 mg twice daily (a medication used in the treatment of leprosy) has been used, but its effectiveness has been questioned. Dapsone was thought to be effective during the early stages of treatment as it works on decreasing the severity of the inflammation caused by the bite toxin. Dapsone has not been included as a routine component in the Wilderness Medical Kit. Prophylactic use of antibiotic has been recommended. Avoid the application of heat to this wound, even though it is inflamed and necrotic.

Give ibuprofen 200 mg 4 tablets every six hours to help with pain and to reduce inflammation. From the Rx Oral/Topical Unit give Decadron 4 mg every 6 hours (your medical kit supply will be exhausted in 2½ days, but it is doubtful that steroid therapy is of benefit after that time). Apply triple antibiotic ointment from the topical bandaging unit and cover with Spenco 2nd Skin dressing.

Early excision of the bite was recommended as the standard of care for this bite, but treatment with antivenin negates the necessity of this approach. Without its availability, early diagnosis is important since many of the above symptoms can be alleviated if the bitten area is literally excised, or cut out. This should be performed during the first 8 hours, ideally by a physician, and only if the diagnosis is certain. Excision should be performed when the necrotic area has grown to .4 inch (1 cm) in size and should extend to include the red, indurated surrounding tissue.

TICKS

More vector-borne diseases are transmitted in the U.S. by ticks than by any other agent (see Table 6). Ticks must have blood meals to survive their various transformations. It is during these meals that disease can be transmitted to humans and other animals. Two families of ticks can transmit disease to humans: the Ixodidae, or hard ticks, and the Argasidae, or soft ticks. The life cycle of the hard ticks takes two years to complete, including the egg, the six-legged larva or seed tick, the eight-legged immature nymph, and the eight-legged mature adult. They must remain attached from hours to days while obtaining their blood meal. Disease will not be transferred if the tick can be removed before 24 hours. The soft ticks can live many years without food. They have several nymphal stages and may take multiple blood meals. They usually stay attached less than 30 minutes. Of the soft ticks, only the genus ornithodoros transmit disease in the U.S., namely relapsing fever. The 24-hour rule does not apply in this case.

Prevention of attachment is the best defense against tick borne disease. DEET insect repellents are very effective against ticks (see page 154). Permethrin 0.5% spray treated clothing kills ticks upon contact. The combination of permethrin on clothing and DEET on skin is 100% effective against tick attachment.

OK, so you didn't follow my advice in the above paragraph and you find a tick attached, how do you remove it? A tried and true method is to grasp the skin around the insertion of the tick with a pair of fine point tweezers and pull straight outward, removing the tick and a chunk of skin. For some reason this doesn't hurt. Hot wires, matches, glue, fingernail polish, Vaseline, all do not work. Burning the tick might cause it to vomit germs right into the victim, yet it will not let go. Be careful not to grasp the tick body—crushing it might also cause germs to be injected into the victim. During 1994 Sawyer Products plans to release a new item called The Tick Plier® which promises to be an effective and painless device for tick removal.

CATERPILLAR REACTIONS

The puss caterpillar (*Megalopyge opercularis*) of the southern U.S. and the gypsy moth caterpillar (*Lymantria dispar*) of the northeastern U.S. have bristles that cause an almost immediate skin rash and welt formation. Treatment includes patting the victim with a piece of adhesive tape to remove these bristles. Further treatment is discussed on page 110.

MILLIPEDE REACTIONS

Millipedes do not bite, but contact can cause skin irritation. Cold packs can reduce discomfort. Wash thoroughly and treat as indicated on page 110.

CENTIPEDE BITES

Some of the larger centipedes can inflict a painful bite that causes a local swelling and painful, red lesion. Treatment with a cold pack is usually sufficient. Some bites are severe and regional lymph node enlargement may occur, which will be a swelling of the nodes generally at the joints along the blood flow pattern towards the heart from the bite site. Swelling at the bite location may persist for weeks. Adequate treatment consists of pain medication and local application of dibucaine ointment. Infiltration of the area with lidocaine 1% from the Rx Injectable Module provides instant relief and is justified in severe cases.

MOSQUITOS

The best mosquito repellent invented to date has been DEET (n,n diethyl-m-toluamide). This product has undergone a revolution in the past 20 years, ranging from the earliest preparations of 12% strength to numerous products marketing 100% DEET concentration. Between 10% to 15% of DEET applied to the skin surface is excreted in the user's urine. This fact, coupled with a few reports of convulsions in children using DEET, indicates that we should probably minimize the total amount placed on the skin. Two approaches are being made to maintain effectiveness of the stronger concentrations with less exposure. One is the use of a polymer formula that keeps the DEET from evaporating or absorbing into the skin as rapidly (such as the 3-M Ultrathion 35% product). The other is the composite based formula system that adds a synergist to enhance the effectiveness of the DEET. Probably the best product on the market at this time is a composite called DEET Plus® made by Sawyer Products. DEET Plus consists of 17.5% DEET, 5% synergist N-octyl bicycloheptene dicarboximide (MGK

Synergist 264), and a black fly repellent, 2% Di-n-propyl Isocinchomeron-ate (MGK Repellent 326). A thin coating of DEET Plus lotion will last for many hours, even under tropical or Arctic conditions. I have used this product during enormous mosquito and black fly exposures and find that it works 6 to 12 hours. This minimizes the number of reapplications and the total DEET exposure tremendously.

I never use 100% DEET. If I was purchasing a 100% DEET product, I would at least cut it with rubbing alcohol by 25% to 50% (the old Army formulation was 75% DEET, 25% alcohol). Without the use of a synergist formula, high concentrations of DEET are necessary for the high insect loads of the Arctic or tropics.

Adequate mosquito netting for the head and for the tent or cot while sleeping is essential. Spraying netting and clothing with .5% pyrethrin (Permone Tick Repellent), increases the effectiveness of the netting and decreases bug bites enormously. Pyrethrin is an insecticide, not a repellent. It kills mosquitos, ticks, black flies, etc., and does not simply chase them away. It must not be applied to the skin.

I have not found Vitamin B1 (thiamine) to be an effective preventative oral agent, but the recommended dose by those who do is 100 mg daily for one week prior to departure and daily thereafter. Electronic sound devices to repel these critters have never dented mosquito buzzing or biting enthusiasm in the far north in my experience, but I have friends who use them enthusiastically (under less obnoxious circumstances).

A considerable number of bites, or sensitivity to bites, may require an antihistamine, such as Benadryl 25 mg capsules every 6 hours from the Non-Rx Oral Medication Module. Dibucaine ointment 1% from the Topical Bandaging Unit, applied every 6 hours, can provide local itch relief.

BLACK FLIES

DEET compounds will work, but the concentration must be 30% or greater and even the pure formula will work only a short time. It is best to use a specific black fly repellent or a composite formula such as the DEET Plus, mentioned in the section on mosquitos.

For years Skin So Soft, a bath oil marketed by your local Avon representative, has been mentioned as a black fly repellent. It does work, but it requires frequent applications, approximately every 15 minutes.

Netting and heavy clothes that can be sealed at the cuffs may be required. All black fly species like to land and crawl, worming their way under and through protective clothing and netting. Spray clothing and netting with .5% pyrethrin as mentioned in the section on mosquitos.

Black fly bites can result in nasty sores which are usually self-limited, although at times slow healing. If infection is obvious, treat as indicated in the section on skin infection on page 108. Dibucaine ointment 1% will provide local pain relief. Benadryl 25 mg every 6 hours will help reduce swelling and itch.

NO-SEE-UMS AND BITING GNATS

These two examples of insect life are the scourge of the North Country, or any country in which they may be found. Many local people refer to any small black fly as a "No-See-Um", but the true bug by that name is indeed very hard to see. They usually come out on a hot, sticky night. The attack is sudden and feels like fire over your entire exposed body surface area. Under the careful examination of a flashlight, you will notice an incredibly small gnat struggling with his head down, merrily chomping away. Make the bug portion of the previous sentence plural please. This is an ideal time for application of the DEET Plus® or you will have to resort to a strong DEET product of 35% or greater. Immersion in cold water will help relieve symptoms temporarily. One remedy for the sting which I understand works quite well, but which I have never had along to try, is an application of Absorbine Jr®!

Gnats, on the other hand, are a small black fly whose bite is seldom felt. But these gentle biters leave behind a red pimple-like lesion to remind you of their visit. A rash of these pimples around the neck and ankles attests to their ability to sneak through protective clothing. Treat severe cases with Benadryl 25 mg every 6 hours. Application of the 1% dibucaine ointment provides local relief.

SCORPION STING

Most North American scorpion stings are relatively harmless. Stings usually cause only localized pain and slight swelling. The wound may feel numb. Benadryl and Percogesic may be all that is required for treatment. A cold pack will help relieve local pain.

The potentially lethal *Centruroides sculptuatus* is the exception to this rule. This yellow colored scorpion lives in Mexico, New Mexico, Southern Utah, Arizona, and the California side of the Colorado River. The sting causes immediate, severe pain with swelling and subsequent numbness. The neurotoxin injected with this bite may cause respiratory failure. Respiratory assistance may be required (see page 20). Tapping on the wound lightly with your finger will cause the patient to withdraw due to severe pain. This is an unusual reaction and does not occur with most insect stings. A specific antivenin is available in Mexico and is also produced by the Poisonous Animals Laboratory at Arizona State University for local use. In addition to the antivenin, atropine may be needed to reduce muscle cramping, blurred vision, hypertension, respiratory difficulty, and excessive salivation. This is not included in the Wilderness Medical Kit. Methocarbamol may be given as described in the section on Black Widow Spider bites (page 151). Narcotics such as Demerol and morphine can increase the toxicity and should be avoided. You may give Percogesic from the Non-Rx Oral Medical Module.

ANT, FIRE ANT
While many ants can alert you to their presence with a burning bite, the latter can produce an intensely painful bite which pales to insignificance due to a surrounding cluster of stings. While holding on tightly with his biting pincer and pivoting around, the ant then stings repeatedly in as many places as the stinger can reach, causing a cluster of small, painful blisters to appear. These can take 8 to 10 days to heal. Treatment is with cold packs and pain medication. Large local reactions may require antihistamine such as the Benadryl 25 mg, 2 capsules every 6 hours and even Decadron 4 mg twice daily. Local application of dibucaine ointment 1% can provide some relief. Treat with pain medication as required.

The greatest danger is to the hypersensitive individual who may have an anaphylactic reaction. This should be treated as indicated under ANAPHYLACTIC SHOCK, page 145.

CATFISH STINGS
Apply hot water as indicated under STING RAY. The wound must be properly cleaned and irrigated using surgical scrub, if available, or soap. Place the patient on oral antibiotic for several days to decrease the chance of wound infection which is common with this injury. Treat infected wound as described on page 108.

SEA URCHIN
Punctures from sea urchin spines cause severe pain and burning. Besides trauma from the sharp spines, some species inject a venom. The wound can

appear red and swollen or even blue to black from a harmless dye which may be contained in the spines. Generalized symptoms are rare, but may include weakness, numbness, muscle cramps, nausea, and occasionally shortness of breath. The spines should be removed thoroughly—a very tedious process. Very thin spines may be absorbed by the body without harm, but some may form a reactive tissue around them (granulomas) several months later. Spines may migrate into joints and cause pain and inhibit movement or lodge against a nerve and cause extreme pain. The discoloration of the dye causes no problems, but may be mistaken for a thin spine. Relief may be obtained by soaking in hot water (110° to 113° F or 43° to 45° C) for 20 to 30 minutes. Vinegar or acetic acid soaks several times a day may help dissolve spines that are not found. Evacuation and treatment by a physician is advisable.

JELLYFISH

Jellyfish tentacles in contact with human skin can cause mild pricking to burning, shooting, terrible pain. The worse danger is shock and drowning. Avoid the use of hot water in treating this injury. First, pour ocean water over the area. Try to remove the tentacles with gloved hands. Pour alcohol (or ideally formalin) over the wound, which will prevent the nematocysts from firing more poison. Both ammonia or vinegar would work, but not as well as formalin or alcohol. Urine may be used, but do not use fresh water. Powder the area with a dry powder such as flour or baking powder. Gently scrape off the mess with a knife, clam shell or other sharp instrument, but avoid cutting the nematocysts with a sharp blade. Apply hydrocortisone 1% cream 4 times daily from the Non-Rx Topical Bandaging Module or Topicort .25% ointment twice daily from the Rx Oral/Topical Module for inflammation.

CORAL STINGS

These injuries are treated as indicated under JELLYFISH.

CORAL CUTS, BARNACLE CUTS

Clean the wound thoroughly—trivial wounds can later flare into real disasters that may go on for years. Scour thoroughly with a coarse cloth or soft brush and surgical scrub or soapy water. Then apply hydrogen peroxide to help bubble out fine particles and bacteria. Apply triple antibiotic ointment from the Non-Rx Topical Bandaging Module. Manage this wound as discussed in the section on laceration care, page 85. If an infection ensues, treat as indicated on page 108.

STING RAY

The damage is done by the barbed tail, which lacerates the skin, imbedding pieces of tail material and venom into the wound. The wound bleeds heavily, pain increases over 90 minutes and takes 6 to 48 hours to abate.

Immediately rinse the wound with sea water and remove any particles of the tail sheath which are visible as these particles continue to release venom. Hot water is the treatment of choice—applied as soon as possible and as hot as the patient can stand it (110°–113° F, 43°–45° C). The heat will destroy the toxin rapidly and remove the pain that the patient is experiencing. After hot water has been applied and all tail particles removed, the wound may be closed with taping techniques (see page 85). Elevation of the wound is important. If particularly dirty, leave the wound open and continue to use intermittent hot soaks as described on page 108. Questionably dirty wounds should be treated with Floxin 400 mg 1 tablet twice daily or doxycycline 100 mg twice daily from the Rx Oral Medication Module. As these are nasty, painful wounds, treat for shock from the onset.

SCORPION FISH

Same treatment as STING RAY.

SPONGE RASH

Sponges handled directly from the ocean can cause an allergic reaction that appears immediately. Fine spicules may also break off in the outer layer of skin also causing inflammation. It will be difficult to tell whether your victim is suffering from the allergic reaction or the spicules, or both. Soak the affected skin by applying vinegar to a cloth and covering for 15 minutes. Dry the skin and pat with the adhesive side of tape to remove sponge spicules. Again soak in vinegar for 5 minutes. An application of rubbing alcohol for 1 minute has been suggested. Then apply hydrocortisone 1% cream 4 times a day from the Non-Rx Topical Bandaging Module or Topicort .25% ointment twice daily from the Rx Oral/Topical Medication Module for several days until the inflammation subsides.

INFECTIOUS DISEASE

Geographical distribution, vector or method of transmission, ability to protect by life style or immunization, and the availability of treatment are the major concerns the outdoors traveler faces with regard to infectious disease. This book emphasizes North American illness and the most likely contagions to afflict adventure travelers to developing countries. It is polite to call Third World countries developing countries, but actually some of them are "undeveloping." In these, many circumstances, including legal as well as medical, are deteriorating. Prior to any trip out of the country, call the U.S. Department of State Advisory Hotline at (202) 647–5225 for the latest information concerning political unrest. This number includes health issues at times. Also call the Centers for Disease Control and Prevention International Travelers' Hotline at (404) 332–4559.[12]

The following table summarizes wilderness related diseases found in Canada and the United States, listing organism and method of transmittal.

TABLE 6		
WILDERNESS DISEASES OF NORTH AMERICA*		
Illness	Mode	Page Number
Babesiosis	tick	162
Blastomycosis	soil	163
Coccidioidomycosis	soil	164
Colorado Tick Fever	tick	164
Echinococcus	water	165
Ehrlichiosis	tick	166
Encephalitis	mosquito	166
Giardiasis	water	167
Hantavirus	rodents/soil	167
Hepatitis A, E	water, food	168
Hepatitis B, C, D	blood, sex	169
Lyme disease	tick	169
Meningococcal meningitis	people	171
Plague	rodents/flea, people	172

*This is not an all inclusive list. Also, many of these diseases have world wide distribution.

Illness	Mode	Page Number
Rabies	mammals	172
Relapsing Fever	tick	173
Rocky Mountain Spotted Fever	tick	174
Tetanus	soil	176
Tick Paralysis	tick	176
Trichinosis	food	176
Tuberculosis	people	178
Tularemia	tick, fly	179
Typhus, endemic	fleas	179

TABLE 7

SIGNIFICANT WILDERNESS DISEASES OF THE WORLD

Illness	Mode	Page Number
Cholera	water	163
Dengue	mosquito	165
Malaria	mosquito	170
Schistosomiasis	snail/water	174
Tapeworms	food/water	175
Trypanosomiasis, African	fly	177
Trypanosomiasis, American	#	177
Typhoid Fever	water/food	26
Typhus, Epidemic	lice	180
Yellow Fever	mosquito	180

#See text for vector description

BABESIOSIS

First discovered in Yugoslavia in 1957 and the U.S. in 1968, this is a malaria-like illness caused by a protozoan parasite that invades red blood cells. Two species have been identified, *Babesia microti* causing disease in the northeastern U.S. and *B. equi* causing disease in California. An unidentified species caused this disease in a patient in Washington State. Over 450 confirmed cases have been reported from the offshore islands of the Northeast, Maryland, Virginia, Georgia, Wisconsin, Minnesota, California, and Washington. Several species of Ixodes ticks transmit babesiosis.

Symptoms gradually begin one week after a tick bite with fatigue and loss of appetite giving way in several days to fever, drenching sweats, muscle ache and headache. The illness ranges from mild to severe, with death occurring in about 10% of patients. Treatment is available with oral quinine plus clindamycin (not included in the recommended medical kit).

BLASTOMYCOSIS

This infectious disease is caused by a fungus, *Blastomyces dermatitidis*. Outbreaks usually cluster with multiple members of a party becoming ill. It is found in the Mississippi River Valley and the southeastern United States. It is also found in various parts of Africa. In the U.S. it has been associated with beaver lodges and in digging contaminated soil. It can also come from dog bites.

Onset of illness is slowly progressive, usually starting with a cough and developing into a pneumonia with fevers, shortness of breath, chest pain, and drenching sweats. Infected blood carries the fungus to the skin and other tissues. Skin lesions enlarge with a collapsed center, purplish–red border and frequent ulcerations.

Antifungal drugs are available, such as oral Ketoconazole, 800 mg given daily. In most untreated patients the disease is slowly progressive and fatal.

CHOLERA

This intestinal infection is caused by a bacterium, *Vibrio cholerae*, which produces profuse, cramping diarrhea. Death can come from dehydration, indeed the death toll can reach the tens of thousands during an epidemic. Ingestion of water contaminated with the bacterium causes spread of the disease. Man is the only documented host for this disease. In the past 20 years cholera has spread from India and Southeast Asia to Africa, the Middle East, and Southern Europe. Since 1991 it has spread to the New World with thousands of cases reported from Peru and many other countries of South and Central America and Mexico. The current vaccine provides such low immunity that its use is not justified. No country officially requires cholera vaccine for entry.

Treatment is with oral rehydration as indicated on page 70. The strain of cholera that is raging in most of the world is very resistant to antibiotics and, fortunately, does not require antibiotic treatment. Imodium 2 mg can be used for symptomatic relief, 2 capsules immediately with an additional capsule after each loose stool.

COCCIDIOIDOMYCOSIS

San Joaquin Fever, Valley Fever

This fungal infection is caused by *Coccidiodes immitis.* Found in the San Joaquin Valley and throughout the southwestern United States. This disease is caught by inhaling the fungal spore in dust.

Symptoms can be delayed in travelers until after leaving the endemic area. The primary symptoms are those of an upper respiratory infection, bronchitis, or a pneumonia. Incubation time is varied and a progressive form may occur weeks, months, or years after the original infection in people with decreased immunity (AIDS patients, people on steroids, or those receiving chemotherapy).

Treatment is not required for those with upper respiratory infection symptoms. The diagnosis should be made with special blood tests to avoid missing other pneumonias that require specific treatment. Progressive disease must be treated with intravenous antifungal medications.

COLORADO TICK FEVER

A viral disease spread by Ixodides (hard-shelled) ticks, this disease is 20 times more common than Rocky Mountain Spotted Fever in Colorado. It is also found in the other states of the Western Rocky Mountains and provinces of Western Canada. It is most frequent in April-May at low altitudes and June-July at high altitudes.

Onset is abrupt, with chills, fever of 100.4° to 104° F (38° to 40° C), muscle ache, headache, eye pain, and eye sensitivity to light (photophobia). The patient feels weak and nauseated, but vomiting is unusual. During the first 2 days, up to 12% of the victims develop a rash. In half the cases the fever disappears after 2 to 3 days and the patient feels well for 2 days. Then a second bout of illness starts which lasts intensely for 2 to 4 days. This second phase subsides with the patient feeling weak for 1 to 2 additional weeks.

This disease requires no treatment other than bed rest, fluids to prevent dehydration, and medications to treat fever and aches. However, as the same ticks can also spread potentially dangerous Rocky Mountain Spotted Fever, treatment with doxycycline (100 mg twice daily) as described in that section should be started immediately and this therapy continued for 14 days. This should be accomplished without waiting for the characteristic rash of Rocky Mountain Spotted Fever or the fever pattern of Colorado Tick Fever to develop or for a firm diagnoses of either to be established by a physician.

DENGUE

Breakbone Fever, Dandy Fever

This viral infection is caused by a virus (Group B arbovirus or flavivirus) and is spread by bites from *Aedes aegypti* mosquito. Dengue is endemic throughout the tropics and subtropics. Check for latest information on active disease areas and countries receptive to this disease by contacting IAMAT for specific country update (see Appendix B).

After an incubation period of 3 to 15 (usually 5 to 8) days, there is a sudden onset of fever (104° F, 40° C), chills, headache, low back ache, pain behind the eyes with movement of the eyes, extreme aching in the legs and joints. The eyes are red and a transient flushing or pale pink rash occurs, mostly on the face. There is a relatively slow pulse rate for the temperature (see page 26). The fever lasts 48 to 96 hours, followed by 24 hours of no fever and a sense of well being. A second rapid temperature increase occurs, but generally not as high as the first. A bright rash spreads from the arms/legs to the trunk, but generally not the face. Palms and soles may be bright red and swollen. There is a severe headache and other body aches as well. The fever, rash, and headache constitute the "dengue triad." The illness lasts for weeks, but mortality is nil. Treatment is rest and the use of pain and fever medication. A condition called Dengue Hemorrhagic Fever Shock Syndrome is lethal and occurs in patients younger than 10 exclusively; generally infants under one year of age. Dengue may be confused with Colorado tick fever, typhus, yellow fever, or other hemorrhagic fevers.

ECHINOCOCCUS

Also called hydatid disease, this infection is caused by the larval stage of a tapeworm found in dogs (with sheep as an intermediate host), or in wilderness areas found in wolves (with moose as the intermediate host). This disease is world-wide, but most commonly a problem in Europe, Russia, Japan, Alaska, Canada, and the continental United States. When ingested by sheep, moose, or humans, the eggs form embryos which pass through the intestinal circulation into the liver and sometimes beyond into the lungs, brain, kidney and other tissue. There a fluid filled cyst forms which contains scolices, brood capsules, and second generation (daughter) cysts containing infectious scolices. The hydatid cysts maintain their presence, sometimes bursting and spreading in a malignant fashion causing destruction of liver, lung and other critical tissues. After remaining without symptoms for decades, abdominal pain, jaundice, or chest pain and coughing may commence.

If the intermediate host is eaten by a carnivore (dog, wolf, or man), the infectious scolices are released into the GI tract where they develop into adult worms and the life cycle continues.

Most hydatid disease is from a particular tapeworm known as *Echinococcus granulosis*, but a rapidly progressive form develops when infection is caused by the *Echinococcus multilocularis* tapeworm. This tape worm is carried primarily by domestic dogs, cats, and by foxes. Multiple small cysts form that multiply rapidly. The result is often fatal. There is no adequate medical treatment, with attempts at surgical removal of multiple cysts being the only reliable hope for cure.

EHRLICHIOSIS

Since its discovery in 1987, more than 250 cases have been reported from 21 states, principally Oklahoma, Missouri, and Georgia. The time of greatest risk is May through July. This is a rickettsial infection caused by *Ehrlichia chafeensis* and is spread by several species of ticks.

The incubation time ranges from 1 to 21 days (mean 7 days). It presents with high fever and headache, with other common symptoms being tiredness, nausea, vomiting, muscle ache, and loss of appetite. Twenty percent of victims develop a rash, but this rash is seldom on the feet or hands. Deaths have occurred.

The drug of choice is doxycycline 100 mg twice daily. The appropriate length of treatment is unknown.

ENCEPHALITIS

Encephalitis from Group A Arbovirus (Western Equine Encephalitis, Eastern Equine Encephalitis, Venezuelan Equine Encephalitis) in Alaska, U.S., and Canada, and Group B Arbovirus (St. Louis Encephalitis) in the U.S. can be prevented by liberal use of repellent and covering exposed areas with netting or clothing to prevent bites from infected mosquitos. Symptoms of these illnesses include high fever (104° F, 40° C) and generally headache, stiff neck and vomiting and, at times, diarrhea. These cases can be fatal and require evacuation to medical help. Cool the patient with external means (cool water, fanning), and the use of aspirin or Mobigesic. The disease occurs in epidemics; be very careful of mosquito exposure when the disease becomes prevalent.

GIARDIASIS

Intestinal infection by *Giardia lamblia*, a single cell parasite, is becoming a significant problem in wilderness travel in the United States and is a very common cause of traveler's diarrhea in the Middle East, India, and the western USSR, particularly the city of Leningrad. The stools of infected individuals contain the infective cyst form of the parasite. These cysts can live in water for longer than 3 months. Other mammalian vectors, such as the beaver, are responsible for much of the wilderness spread of this disease.

In the active disease, the trophozoite form attaches to the small bowel by means of a central sucker. Multiplication is by binary fission, or division. Approximately 2 weeks after ingestion of the cysts there is either a gradual or abrupt onset of persistent watery diarrhea which usually resolves in 1 to 2 weeks, but which may persist less severely for several months. Abdominal pain, bloating, nausea, and weight loss from malabsorption may occur. Giardiasis is often without symptoms at all and a chronic carrier state exists. In the U.S. about 4% of stools submitted for parasitology examination contain *G. lamblia* cysts.

Diagnosis is by finding cysts in stools or trophozoites from gastric suction or the "string test" from the duodenum. This later test is performed by having the patient swallow a string, allowing the far end to pass into the first part of the bowel, or duodenum. When the string is pulled out, a microscopic examination may demonstrate the presence of trophozoites. In active disease the cysts are routinely secreted, but in the chronic carrier state repeated stool examinations (at least three) are required to provide a 95% accuracy of test results.

Treatment is with one of several drugs available in the U.S., the most commonly used being Flagyl (metronidazole) 250 mg 3 times daily for 5 days. A better drug, but not available in the U.S., is quinacrine 100 mg 3 times daily for 5 days. Prevention is by proper filtration of water, adequate chemical treatment, or heating water to 150° F (66° C). See page 71 for a full discussion of water treatment.

HANTAVIRUS

This virus was the cause of death amongst members of the Navaho Indian Nation in New Mexico in 1993. The virus has been identified in serum samples from 42 people in 12 states with the greatest concentration in southwestern United States. It is caught by inhaling dust contaminated with feces from an infected deer mouse (*Peromyscus maniculatus*).

The onset of illness is a period of fever, muscle ache, and cough, followed by an abrupt onset of acute respiratory distress. The mortality rate has been 60%! There is no specific treatment available. Avoiding breathing dust which may contain the contaminated mouse feces is the preventative measure.

HEPATITIS A (INFECTIOUS HEPATITIS)

A viral infection of the liver, this disease is wordwide in distribution. It is transmitted by ingestion of infected feces, either through water supplies contaminated by human sewage, food handled by persons with poor hygiene, or contaminated food such as raw shellfish grown in impure water. Contaminated milk, even infusion of infected blood products (see Hepatitis B), can spread this disease.

The period from the time of exposure to the appearance of symptoms takes 15 to 50 days. The disease can range from minor flu-like symptoms to fatal liver disease. Most cases resolve favorably within 6 to 12 weeks. Symptoms start abruptly with fever, lethargy, and nausea. Occasionally a rash develops. A characteristic loss of taste for cigarettes is frequent. In 3 to 10 days the urine turns dark, followed by jaundice - or yellowing of the whites of the eyes and the skin. The stool may turn light colored. There is frequently itching and joint pain. The jaundice peaks within one to two weeks and fades during the two to four week recovery phase. The hepatitis A patient stops shedding virus in the stool prior to the jaundice developing, and is therefore not contagious by the time the diagnosis is normally made. Personal hygiene helps prevent this spread, but isolation of the patient is not strictly required.

In most cases no specific treatment is required. After a few days to 2 weeks appetite generally returns and bed confinement is no longer required, even though jaundice still remains. The best guideline is the disappearance of the lethargy and feeling of illness that appeared in the first stages of the disease. Restrictions of diet have no value, but a low fat diet is generally more palatable. If profound prostration occurs, and certainly when feasible, the trip should be terminated for the patient and he should be placed under medical care. If possible, contacts should receive Gamma–globulin 0.02 ml/kg IM. The use of Gamma–globulin prophylactically is discussed in Appendix B.

HEPATITIS B

(Serum Hepatitis)

A different viral infection of the liver, this disease is also world-wide in distribution. Transmission is primarily through infusion of infected blood products, sexual contact, use of contaminated needles, syringes, or even sharing contaminated razor blades. Dental procedures, acupuncture, ear piercing, and tattooing with contaminated equipment will also spread this disease.

Incubation period from time of exposure to the development of symptoms is longer than with hepatitis A, namely 30 to 180 days. The symptoms are similar, but the onset is less abrupt and the incidence of fever is lower. There is a greater chance of developing chronic hepatitis (5% to 10% of cases). Mortality is higher, especially in elderly patients where it ranges from 10% to 15%.

Immunization is available and is very effective (see Appendix B).

HEPATITIS C

(Non-A, Non-B)

A form of hepatitis, with similar manifestations to Hepatitis B, has been designated as Hepatitis C (formerly "Non-A, Non-B" since blood tests for evidence of exposure to those virus particles was not previously found). The transmission is probably the same as for Hepatitis B. Incubation period is from less than 2 weeks, to more than 25 weeks, with an average of 7 weeks for the development of clinical disease. There is no specific treatment.

HEPATITIS D

Hepatitis D, or the "delta agent" can only infect a person who has Hepatitis B. The presence of this mutated RNA particle causes the infection to be more fulminant. It spreads only by contaminate needle use.

HEPATITIS E

An epidemic form of Hepatitis (that is not A) has been termed Hepatitis E. There may be several viruses that are involved. Spread is primarily through contaminated food or water. The incubation period from time of contact ranges from 2 to 25 weeks. The disease mimics Hepatitis A.

LYME DISEASE

Lyme disease is caused by a spirochete, *Borrelia burgdorferi*. The disease lives in various mammals, but is transmitted to humans by the bite of several species of ticks. The disease is most common in the Northeast, extending through Connecticut and Massachusetts down to Maryland; in Wisconsin and Minnesota; throughout the states of California and Oregon; in various south Atlantic and south central states; with cases reported from 43 of the lower 48 states. It is located across the USSR, in China, Australia, Japan and in several European countries.

The disease goes through several phases. In Stage One, after an incubation of 3 days to a month, probably 95% of victims develop a circular lesion in the area of the bite. It has a clear to pink center, raised border, is painless, and ranges from 1 to 23 inches in diameter. There are usually several such patches. The patient feels lethargic, has headache, muscle and joint pain, and enlarged lymph nodes. In Stage Two 10% to 15% of patients can develop a meningitis, less than 10% develop heart problems. Symptoms may last for months, but are generally self-limited. Approximately 60% enter Stage Three - the development of actual arthritis. Frequently a knee is involved. The swelling can be impressive. Stage Three can start abruptly several weeks to 2 years after the onset of the initial rash.

Treatment of Stage One Lyme disease is tetracycline, such as doxycycline 100 mg taken twice daily for 20 days. Alternate drugs are penicillin and erythromycin. Treatment of choice for Stage Two and Three Lyme disease consists of Rocephin 2 gram given IV daily for 14 to 21 days.

One possible manifestation of Lyme disease is the development of a facial paralysis on one side called Bell's Palsy. The involved side is expressionless with the patient being unable to move the muscles of the forehead, around the eye, or the face. While there are other causes of Bell's Palsy, in North America this problem must be considered as Lyme Disease until ruled out by a physician. Treatment of Bell's Palsy caused by Lyme disease is with oral antibiotic for 21 days.

MALARIA

Human malaria is caused by four species of a protozoa: *Plasmodium falciparum, P. vivax, P. ovale,* and *P. malariae.* The infection is acquired from the bite of an infected female Anopheles mosquito. It may also be spread by blood transfusion. Falciparum malaria is the most serious. While all forms of this disease make people ill and may be lethal, this is the one that most often kills.

Regions of the world where malaria may be acquired are sub— Saharan Africa, parts of Mexico and Central America, Haiti, parts of South America, the Middle East, the Indian subcontinent and Southeast Asia. The mainstay of *P. falciparum* prevention has been Aralen (chloroquine) 500 mg, 1 tablet every week starting one week before departure, continuing during the trip, and for 6 weeks after returning. Resistance to chloroquine by the deadly *P. falciparum* has become widespread. For travelers in resistant areas the current prophylactic medication is Larium (mefloquine) 250 mg 1 tablet weekly, starting 1 week prior to departure and continuing for 4 weeks after return. Persons traveling to remote malarious areas should also consider taking 3 tablets of the drug Fansidar (pyrimethamine-sulfadoxine) for consumption at one time as a presumptive treatment in case the symptoms of malaria develop (ache, fever, or any questionable flu-like symptoms). This person should also seek medical help as soon as possible. Persons with a sulfa allergy may not take this drug. An alternate drug regimen, especially necessary when *P. falciparum* becomes resistant to mefloquine is the use of doxycycline 100 mg to be taken once daily for prevention.

In areas with relapsing malaria (*P. vivax* and *P. ovale*), primaquine should be taken 1 tablet daily during the last 2 weeks of chloroquine therapy. This is usually appropriate for those with long exposure in areas with a high concentration of these strains of malaria. IAMAT literature on malaria (see Appendix C) provides the percentage of *P. falciparum* vs *P. vivax* and *P. ovale* as well as current information on resistance to chloroquine for each country.

MENINGOCOCCAL MENINGITIS

This acute bacterial infection causes inflammation in linings of the brain and central nervous system. Many cases are without symptoms or consist of a mild upper respiratory illness. Severe cases begin with sudden fever, sore throat, chills, headache, stiff neck, nausea, and vomiting. Within 24 to 48 hours the victim becomes drowsy, mentally confused, followed by convulsions, coma, and death. Immediate and appropriately large doses of the proper antibiotic are critical to save the patient's life (the Wilderness Medical Kit only has Rocephin which must be given in large amounts, 1 or 2 grams IM twice daily). The disease is spread by contact with the nasal secretions of infected persons (sneezing and coughing).

While the disease is found worldwide, large epidemics are more common in tropical countries, especially sub-Saharan Africa in the dry season, New Delhi (India), and in Nepal.

In 80% of healthy young adults bacterial meningitis is caused by meningococci, discussed above, or pneumococci. Vaccines are available against both of these organisms (see Appendix B).

PLAGUE

Plague is caused by a bacterium (*Yersinia pestis*) that infects wild rodents in many parts of the world, including the western United States and parts of South America, Africa, and Asia. Epidemics occur when domestic rats become infected and spread the disease to man. Bubonic plague is transmitted by infected fleas, while pneumonic plague is spread directly to other people by coughing. Plague is accompanied by fever, enlarged lymph nodes (bubonic plague) and less commonly pneumonia (pneumonic plague). Treatment is with doxycycline 100 mg twice daily. Treat fever as necessary. Isolate patient, particularly if coughing. Drainage of abscesses (buboes) may be necessary (see page 108). Exposed persons should be watched for 10 days, but incubation is usually 2 to 6 days. Only travelers to Vietnam, Cambodia, and Laos are at enough risk to consider using plague vaccine, unless a local epidemic has broken out (see Appendix B).

RABIES

Rabies can be transmitted on the North American continent by several species of mammals, namely skunk, bat, fox, coyote, raccoon, bobcat, and wolf. Obviously, if removing an animal from a trap, jogging past an animal, separating mother from child, or taking food from a critter causes an attack, the most likely cause is not rabies. An attack by a wounded animal is cause for concern, as the animal may be wounded due to loss of coordination from rabies. Any unprovoked attack by one of these mammals should be considered an attack by a rabid animal. Dogs and cats in the United States have a low incidence of rabies. Information from local departments of health will indicate if rabies is currently of concern in these animals. Animals whose bites have never caused rabies in humans in the U.S. are livestock (cattle, sheep, horse), rabbit, gerbil, chipmunk, squirrel, rat, and mouse. A significant epidemic of raccoon rabies has now extended from Florida to Connecticut, with isolated reports from New Hampshire and Ohio showing an expansion of this epidemic north and west. Hawaii is the only rabies free state.

In the United States there have been 18 human deaths from rabies reported between 1980 and 1993, 8 of which were acquired during foreign travel. In India 40,000 to 50,000 people die yearly from rabies, with a large incidence in the other developing counties of Asia, Africa, and Latin America.

In many foreign countries the bite of a cat or dog should be considered rabid. Countries free of rabies are England, Australia, Japan, and parts of the Caribbean. In Europe the red fox is the animal most often rabid with documented cases spreading to dogs, cats, cattle, and deer. Canada's rabies occurs mostly in foxes and skunks in the province of Ontario. Mongoose rabies is found in South Africa and the Caribbean islands of Cuba, Puerto Rico, Hispaniola, and Grenada.

The treatment for rabies is prophylaxis with Rabies Immune Globulin 20 IU/kg with half infiltrated around the wound and the remaining half in the gluteal area (upper outer quadrant of the bottom) and human diploid cell vaccine (HDCV) 1 ml given IM in the shoulder on days 0, 3, 7, 14, and 28. The incubation period in a human is 1 to 2 months. Rabies is a vicious disease that is fatal once it clinically develops. Because of this, there is generous use of rabies vaccine and immune globulin. Approximately 28,000 people are vaccinated here yearly to prevent this disease. Persons having to work with potentially rabid animal populations can be immunized with the vaccine and given yearly booster shots. It is possible to obtain the disease by merely being contaminated with the saliva or blood of an infected animal if it comes in contact with a break in the skin or mucous membranes - possibly even by breathing in dust infected with the virus (two cases of human rabies have been attributed to airborne exposures in a bat cave in Texas).[13]

RELAPSING FEVER

This bacterial infection is caused by several species of Borrelia spirochete and is spread by body lice in Asia, Africa and Europe, or by soft body ticks in the Americas (including the western United States), Asia, Africa and Europe. Several cases have been contracted near Spokane, Washington, during the last couple of years.

Symptoms occur 3 to 11 days from contact with the tick or louse vector and start with an abrupt onset of chills, headache, muscular pains and sometimes vomiting. A rash may appear and small hemorrhages present under the skin surface. The fever remains high from 3 to 5 days, then clears suddenly. After 1 to 2 weeks a somewhat milder relapse begins. Jaundice is more common during relapse. The illness again clears, but 2 to 10 similar episodes reoccur at intervals of 1 to 2 weeks until immunity fully develops.

Antibiotic is available for effective treatment. Mortality is low, generally 0–5% in healthy adults. Treatment is with doxycycline 100 mg twice daily for 5 to 10 days. Personal hygiene is effective in preventing louse borne disease, while control of ticks with insect repellent and frequent body checks and tick removal minimize the chance of tick borne disease.

ROCKY MOUNTAIN SPOTTED FEVER

This is an acute and serious infection caused by a microorganism called *Rickettsia rickettsii* and transmitted by Ixodides (hard-shelled) ticks. It is most common in the states of North Carolina, Virginia, Maryland, the Rocky Mountain States, and the state of Washington. The peak incidence of cases is from May to September.

Onset of infection is abrupt, after a 3 to 12-day incubation period (average 7 days from the tick bite). Fever reaches 103° to 104° F (40° C) within two days. There is considerable headache, chills, and muscle pain at the onset. In four days a rash appears on wrists, ankles, soles, palms, and then spreads to the trunk. Initially pink, this rash turns to dark blotches and even ulcers in severe cases.

Any suspected case of Rocky Mountain Spotted Fever should be considered a MEDICAL EMERGENCY. Do not wait for the rash to develop, rather start the patient on the antibiotic from the Rx kit. Give doxycycline 100 mg, 1 tablet every 12 hours and keep on this dosage schedule for 14 days. This is a drug of choice and its early use can cut the death rate from 20% to nearly zero. Prevention is by the careful removal of ticks, the use of insect repellent and protective clothing.

SCHISTOSOMIASIS

(Bilharziasis, Blood Flukes, Safari Fever)
Blood trematodes or flukes are responsible for this disease. The eggs are deposited in fresh water and hatch into motile miracidia which infect snails. After development in the snails, active cercariae emerge which penetrate exposed human skin. Swimming, wading, or drinking fresh water must be avoided in infected areas.

Schistosoma mansoni is found in tropical Africa, part of Venezuela, several Caribbean islands, the Guianas, Brazil and the Middle East. *S. japonicum* is encountered in China, Japan, the Philippines, and Southeast Asia. *S. haematobium* is in Africa, the Middle East, and small portions of India and islands in the Indian Ocean. The former two species are excreted in the stools and the latter in urine. Shedding may occur for years. No isolation is required of patients. Specific treatments for the various species are available. Check for latest information on dangerous areas by contacting IAMAT, the International Medical Assistance for Travellers (see Appendix C).

Initial penetration of the skin causes a itchy rash. After entry, the organism enters the blood stream, migrates through the lungs, and eventually lodges in the blood vessels draining either the gut or the bladder, depending upon the species. While the worms are maturing the victim will have fever, lethargy, cough, rash, abdominal pain, and frequently nausea. In acute infections caused by *S. mansoni* and *S. japonicum*, victims develop a mucoid, bloody diarrhea and tender liver enlargement. Chronic infection leads to fibrosis of the liver with distention of the abdomen. In *S. haematobium* infections the bladder becomes inflamed and eventually fibrotic. Symptoms include painful urination, urgency, blood in urine, and pelvic pain.

TAPEWORMS

Three species of tapeworms infect humans, *Taenia saginata* larvae found in beef, *Taenia solium* in pork, and *Diphyllobothrium latum* in fish. In all three the human ingests undercooked flesh of the host animal acquiring the infective cysts.

The beef tapeworm can be huge, forming lengths of 10 to 30 feet inside the human host. It is common in Mexico, South America, Eastern Europe, the Middle East, and Africa. Symptoms can include stomach pain, weight loss, and diarrhea, but frequently the human host has no clue of the infestation.

The pork tapeworm infests South America, Eastern Europe, Russia and Asia. Generally without symptoms, at times vague abdominal complaints are noted. A complication of this disease is cystocercosis. In this condition the tapeworm larvae penetrate the human intestinal wall, because the human drank water infected with the larvae, and invade body tissues, frequently skeletal muscle and the brain. There they mature into cystic masses. After several years the cysts degenerate and produce local inflammatory reactions that can then cause convulsions, visual problems, or mental disturbances. In this case, the human replaces the pig in the maturation cycle of the tapeworm and it is the human flesh which is contaminated by the tapeworm cyst. This is an unlucky break for the involved human and any cannibal whom he might meet. Any water filtration or purification system can prevent cystocercosis.

Fish tapeworm occurs worldwide, but is particularly a hazard in Scandinavia and the Far East. A single tapeworm, usually without symptoms, results. The worm's absorption of Vitamin B-12 may cause the development of pernicious anemia in the host.

TETANUS

Caused by a bacterium, *Clostridium tetani*, that is located worldwide, most cases occur from very minor wounds such as blisters or even paper cuts rather than rusty barbed wire as so many people seem to think. Onset is gradual, with an incubation period of 2 to 50 (usually 5 to 10) days. The earliest symptom is stiffness of the jaw, with subsequent symptoms developing that include sore throat, stiff muscles, headache, low grade fever, and muscle spasm. As the disease progresses, the patient is unable to open his jaw and the facial muscles may be fixed in a smile with elevated eyebrows. Painful generalized spasms of muscles occur with minor disturbances such as drafts, noise, or someone jarring their bed. Death from loss of respiratory muscle function, or even unknown causes, may ensue. The disease is frequently fatal.

Prevention is obtained by adequate immunization (see Appendix B). A case of tetanus occurred to a hiker on the Appalachian Trail, caught through inadequate immunization and a blister on his heel.

TICK PARALYSIS

Five species of tick in North America produce a neurotoxin in their saliva that can paralyze its victims. Most cases are from the Pacific Northwest and the Rocky Mountain states, and from seven southern states. Spring and summer are the times of highest risk.

The toxin is usually carried by an engorged, pregnant tick. Symptoms begin from 2 to 7 days after the tick begins feeding. Throughout the ordeal the patient's mental function is usually spared. Symptoms start as weakness in the legs which progressively ascends until the entire body is paralyzed over several hours to days. At times the condition presents as ataxia (loss of coordination) without muscle weakness.

The diagnosis is made by finding an embedded tick. After removing the tick, symptoms resolve in hours to days, rarely longer. Untreated tick paralysis can be fatal with mortality rates of 10% to 12%.

TRICHINOSIS

Trichinosis is caused by eating improperly cooked meat infected with the cysts of this parasite. It is most common in pigs, bears (particularly Polar bears) and some marine mammals. Nausea and diarrhea or intestinal cramping may appear within 1 to 2 days, but it generally takes 7 days after indigestion. Swelling of the eyelids is very characteristic on the 11th day.

Afterwards, muscle soreness, fever, pain in the eyes and subconjunctival hemorrhage (see page 44) develop. If enough contaminated food is ingested this can be a fatal disease. Most symptoms disappear in 3 months. Treatment is with pain medication (Percogesic from the Non-Rx Oral Medication Module or Lorcet 10/650 from the Rx Oral Medication Module. The use of steroids such as Decadron (20 mg/day for 3 or 4 days, followed by reduced dosage over the next 10 days) is indicated in severe cases. Thiabendazole is a specific drug for use in this condition, given orally in doses of 25 mg/kg of body weight twice daily for 5 to 10 days. The best prevention is cooking suspected meat at 150° F (66° C) for 30 minutes for each pound of meat.

AFRICAN SLEEPING SICKNESS

(African Trypanosomiasis)

Two species of trypanosomes cause this disease which is transmitted by the bite of the tsetse fly. The severity of the disease depends upon the species encountered. The infection is confined to the area of Africa between 15 degrees north and 20 degrees south of the equator—the exact distribution of the tsetse fly. Man is the only reservoir of *Trypanosoma gambiense* found in West and Central Africa, while wild game is the principle reservoir of *T. rhodesiense* of East Africa.

T. gambiense infection starts with a nodule or a chancre that appears briefly at the site of a tsetse fly bite. Generalized illness appears months to years later and is characterized by lymph node enlargement at the back of the neck and intermittent fever. Months to years after this development invasion of the central nervous system may occur, noted by behavioral changes, headache, loss of appetite, back ache, hallucinations, delusions, and sleeping. In *T. rhodesiense* infection the generalized illness begins 5 to 14 days after the nodule or chancre develops. It is much more intense than the gambian variety and may include acute central nervous system and cardiac symptoms, fever, and rapid weight loss. It has a high rate of mortality. If untreated, death usually occurs within one year.

CHAGAS' DISEASE

(American Trypanosomiasis)

The disease caused by *Trypanosoma cruzi*, a protozoan hemoflagellate, is transmitted through the feces of a brown insect called the "kissing bug" or "assassin bug" in North America. This bug is a member of the Reduviidae family. A name popular in South America is "vinchuca" derived from a word which means "one who lets himself fall down." These bugs live in palm trees, thatching in native huts, and like to drop on their victims while sleeping, frequently biting them on the face or exposed arms. Bitten patients rub the feces into the bite site, thus causing the innoculaton of the infectious agent. This disease is located in parts of South and Central America. Check for latest information on dangerous areas by contacting IAMAT, the International Medical Assistance for Travellers (see Appendix C). At first this disease may have no symptoms. A "chagoma" or red nodule develops at the site of the original infection. This area may then lose its pigmentation. After 1 to 2 weeks, a firm swelling of one eyelid occurs, known as Romana's sign. The swelling becomes purplish in color, lymph node swelling in front of the ear on the same side may occur. In a few days a fever develops, with generalized lymph node swelling. Rapid heart rate, spleen and liver enlargement, swelling of the legs, and meningitis or encephalitis may occur. Serious conditions also can include acute heart failure. In most cases, however, the illness subsides in about 3 months and the patient appears to be living a normal life. The disease continues, however, slowly destroying the heart until 10 to 20 years later chronic congestive heart failure becomes apparent. The underlying cause may never be known, especially in a traveler who has left the endemic area. In some areas of Brazil, the disease attacks the colon, causing flaccid enlargement with profound constipation. This disease is a leading cause of death in South America, generally due to heart failure. As many as 15 million people in South America may be infected. Special blood tests are available through State Boards of Health and Centers for Disease Control. Supportive treatment is given during acute disease and specific treatments are being developed.

TUBERCULOSIS

This infection is caused by one of two bacteria, *Mycobacterium tuberculosis* or *M. bovis*. It results in a very chronic illness than can reactivate many years after it has been apparently killed. In the United States there are 20,000 new cases, with 1,800 deaths yearly. Worldwide there are 8 to 10 million new cases, with 2 to 3 million deaths yearly. This disease is spread primarily by inhalation of infected droplets. The disease also spreads by drinking infected milk or dairy products such as butter.

Active disease usually develops within a year of contact. The early symptoms of fever, night sweats, lethargy, and weight loss can be so gradual that they are initially ignored. Tuberculosis usually infects the lungs, but it can spread throughout the body causing neurological damage, bone infections, and overwhelming infection. Diagnosis is usually made with a chest x-ray which has characteristic findings. A traveler heading into an area with epidemic tuberculosis should have a pre- and post-trip TB skin test. A negative TB skin test does not exclude a diagnosis of TB, but it can be a very useful aid in evaluating the chance that a traveler has contacted tuberculosis. A TB test should be repeated about 6 months after the return to provide adequate chance for it to react. Specific antibiotic therapy is available.

TULAREMIA
(Rabbit Fever; Deer Fly Fever)

This disease can be contracted through exposure to ticks, deer flies, or mosquitos. It is also possible to have cuts infected when working with the pelts, or eating improperly cooked infected rabbits. Similarly, muskrats, foxes, squirrels, mice and rats can spread the disease via direct contact with the carcasses. Stream water may become contaminated by these animals.

An ulcer appears when a wound is involved and lymph nodes become enlarged first in nearby areas and then throughout the body. Pneumonia normally develops. The disease lasts 4 weeks in untreated cases. Mortality in treated cases is almost zero, while in untreated cases it ranges from 6% to 30%.

Treatment of choice is streptomycin, but doxycycline suggested for the Rx Oral/Topical Medication Module works extremely well. The average adult would require an initial dose of 2 tablets, followed by 1 tablet every 12 hours. Continue therapy for 5 to 7 days after the fever has broken.

ENDEMIC TYPHUS, FLEA-BORNE

This disease is also known as murine typhus, rat-flea typhus, New World typhus, Malaya typhus, and urban typhus. This is one of several diseases caused by rickettsia, which resemble both virus and bacteria. Other diseases caused by this order are Rocky Mountain spotted fever, Q-fever, trench fever, and the various typhus diseases. Endemic typhus is due to *Rickettsia typhi*. It is located worldwide, including the southern Atlantic and Gulf coast states of the United States. It is spread to humans through infected rat flea feces.

After an incubation period of 6 to 18 days (mean 10), shaking chills, fever, and headache develops. A rash forms primarily on the trunk, but fades fairly rapidly. The fever lasts about 12 days. This is a mild disease and fatalities are rare. Antibiotic treatment with doxycycline 100 mg given twice daily is very effective. Prevention is directed toward vector (rat and flea) control.

EPIDEMIC TYPHUS, LOUSE-BORNE

This malady is also called classic typhus, European typhus, and jail fever. This disease killed 3 million people during World War II. On the positive side, no American traveler has contracted this disease since 1950. It is most likely to be encountered in mountainous regions of Mexico, Central and South America, the Balkans, eastern Europe, Africa, and many countries of Asia. The causative agent is Rickettsia prowazekii, which is transmitted by infected lice.

Following a 7 to 14 day incubation period, there is a sudden onset of high fever (104° F, 40° C) which remains at a high level, with a usual morning decrease, for about 2 weeks. There is an intense headache. A light pink rash appears on the 4th to 6th day, soon becoming dark red. There is low blood pressure, pneumonia, mental confusion, and bruising in severe cases. Mortality is rare in children less than 10 years of age, but may reach greater than 60% in those over 50. Antibiotics, such as doxycycline 100 mg twice daily, are very effective if given early in the disease. Prevention is proper hygiene and delousing when needed. A vaccine was formerly made in the United States, but is no longer available and is not needed due to the low incidence observed in American travelers.

YELLOW FEVER

An arbovirus, this disease is found in tropical areas of South and Central America and Africa. This viral disease is contracted by the bite of the *Aedes aegypti* mosquito (and other species) two weeks previously. Onset is sudden with a fever of 102° to 104° F (40° C). The pulse is usually rapid the first day, but becomes slow by the second day. In mild cases the fever falls by crises 2 to 5 days after onset. This remission lasts for hours to several days. Next the fever returns, but the pulse remains slow. Jaundice, vomiting of black blood, and severe loss of protein in the urine (causing it to become foamy) occurs during this stage. Hemorrhages may be noted in the mouth and skin (petechiae). The patient is confused and senses are dulled. Delirium, convulsions and coma occur at death in approximately 10% of cases. If the patient is to survive, this last febrile episode lasts from 3 to 9 days. With remission the patient is well, with no after effects from the disease.

Immunization is available and required for travel to many countries (see Appendix B).

ENVIRONMENTAL INJURIES

While ankle sprains, blisters, and diarrhea are the most common problems facing the wilderness traveler,[14] the environmental injuries pose the most likely threat to life (other than the highway system used to reach the trail head).

Foremost amongst these dangers is hypothermia. Death from heat exposure is still the second leading cause of death amongst high school athletes (again discounting the highway and someone killing them for their Starter-Jackets). Unless you live right on the Pacific Coast, lightning can do more than scare you. And for the many of us traveling vertically, the high altitude illnesses are potentially miserable or even lethal experiences.

TABLE 8

THE ENVIRONMENTAL INJURIES

HYPOTHERMIA

The term "hypothermia" refers to the lowering of the body's core temperature to 95° F (35° C); "profound hypothermia" is a core temperature lower than 90° F (32° C). Another important point is that in the wilderness setting, the term "hypothermia" applies to two distinctly different diseases. One is "chronic hypothermia," the slow onset hypothermia of the outdoors traveler exposed to conditions too cold for their equipment to adequately protect them; the other is "acute," or "immersion hypothermia," the rapid onset hypothermia of a person immersed in cold water.

In acute hypothermia, when the onset of the cold core takes less than two hours, the body does not have the time to adapt to the complex physiological responses which it is able to do given more time. In chronic hypothermia, defined as taking six hours or longer to arrive at the cold core, the responses are quite dramatic and include profound dehydration, exhaustion, and complex chemical changes in the blood. The ideal treatment is quite different in the hospital setting, but in the field our treatment options are reduced to basic techniques of preventing further heat loss and some passive reheating maneuvers.[15]

CHRONIC HYPOTHERMIA

It does not have to be bitter cold out to die of hypothermia. In fact most chronic hypothermia deaths occur in the 30° F (0° C) to 50° F (10° C) range. This temperature range places almost all of North America in a high risk status all year long. The essential aspects of surviving this situation are: being prepared to prevent it, recognizing it if it occurs, and knowing how to treat it. Dampness and wind are the most devastating factors to be considered. Dampness as it can reduce the insulation of clothing and cause evaporative heat loss. Wind as the increased convection heat loss can readily strip away body energy, the so called "wind chill" effect.

Factors important in preventing hypothermia are a high level of pre-trip physical conditioning, adequate nutritional and hydration status of trip members, avoiding exhaustion, and availability of adequate insulation. There is increased risk of hypothermia in case of injury, especially shock, or if the above preventative conditions are inadequate.

An initial response to cold is vasoconstriction, or the clamping down of surface blood vessels. This prevents heat from being conducted to the surface by the blood and effectively increases the mantle, or outer layer depth, thus providing an increased insulation layer. If a person becomes profoundly hypothermic, with a core temperature below 90° F, they have concentrated their blood volume into a small inner core. The amount of dehydration in these persons can be profound, approaching 5.5 liters in a person below 90° F—or equivalent to the entire circulatory volume. Of course this fluid loss comes from not only the vascular space, but also fluid from between the cells and within the cells as the body slowly adjusts to the continuing heat loss by shrinking the blood volume in the core and increasing the effective depth of the mantle layer. This causes problems with the rewarming process as a sudden rewarming can lead to "rewarming shock." Hospital methods of rewarming must be coupled with tight metabolic control by adjusting blood factors such as clotting, electrolytes, blood sugar levels, etc. Loss of tight control can occur more easily if a person is rewarmed too rapidly.

In chronic hypothermia rewarming shock and loss of metabolic control is the cause of death, not the so-called "after-drop" phenomenon. After-drop, or the further lowering of core temperature after rewarming has started, is due to the combination of conduction equilibration of heat and a circulation component. By far the most important aspect is the conduction equilibration. This physical property of conduction results in an equilibration of thermal mass as the higher warmth of the core leaches into the colder mantle layer. The amount of after-drop that occurs is dependent upon the rate of cooling that was occurring prior to the rewarming process, not the method of rewarming!

The treatment of the chronic hypothermic victim is to prevent further loss of heat and this generally means providing shelter or more adequate clothing. The victim is exhausted and thus requires rest and food. They are dehydrated and require fluids. If the victim can stand, a roaring fire can provide adequate, controlled heat. Since chronic hypothermia victims are exhausted they will not be able to exercise themselves to warmth. Exercise is a method of generating heat, as is shivering, but when energy stores are consumed, the exhaustion commences and significant hypothermia will begin unless further heat loss is stopped.

Deepening hypothermia will lead to a semi-comatose state and worse. This victim needs to be evacuated to help. Wrap to prevent further heat loss and transport. Chemical heat packs, etc., can be added to the wrap to help offset further heat loss, but care must be taken not to burn the victim. If evacuation is not feasible, heat will have to be added slowly to avoid rewarming shock. Huddling the victim with two rescuers in an adequate sleeping bag may be the only alternative. On all of my expeditions into northern Canada in the winter, we always carry a set of semi-rectangular bags that can twin so that such a rescue is feasible.

ACUTE HYPOTHERMIA

After-drop is, however, a problem in the "acute" or "immersion hypothermic" who has had a significant exposure to cold water. As a rule of thumb, a person who has been in water of 50° (10° C) or less for a period of 20 minutes or longer, is suffering from a severe amount of heat loss. That individual's thermal mass has been so reduced that they are in potentially serious condition. They should not be allowed to move around as this will increase the blood flow to their very cold skin and facilitate a profound circulatory induced after-drop; one that is so great as to be potentially lethal. If this same person is simply wrapped as a litter case and not provided outside heat, there is a real danger of them cooling below a lethal level due to this profound amount of heat loss. The ideal treatment is rapid rewarming of the acute hypothermic by placing them in hot water (110° F/43° C) to allow rapid replacement of heat. These people may have an almost normal core temperature initially, but one that is destined to drop dramatically as their body equilibrates their heat store from their core to their very cold mantle. A roaring fire can be a life saver. If not available, huddling two rescuers with the victim in a large sleeping bag may be the only answer - the same therapy that might have to be employed in the field treatment of chronic hypothermia under some conditions.

The person who has been immersed for less than 20 minutes in cold water can do anything he wants to rewarm. He can run around like crazy, stand by a fire, or just wrap up in warm, dry insulation. The total body thermal mass is still high enough that the temperature equilibration by both the conductive and circulatory components will not reduce the core temperature to a dangerous level.

In review, the person who has been in cold water longer than 20 minutes has experienced such a profound heat loss, that allowing him run around or to even wrap him without additional significant heat will cause a tremendous drop in his core temperature, into a lethal range. And the person who is fished out of the cold water two hours or longer must be considered as approaching chronic hypothermia. He has survived long enough that his physiological protective mechanisms have resulted in dehydration and other changes that are so complex that rapid rewarming can result in rewarming shock and death.

COLD WATER SUBMERSION

Cold water submersion[16] is always associated with asphyxiation andsimultaneous hypothermia. The asphyxiation results in brain death so that prompt rescue and immediate implementation of CPR play an important role in the survival of the victim. Total submersion in cold water results in rapid core cooling which results in a lower oxygen demand by the brain and other body tissues and increases the chance of survival over that of a victim of warm water submersion. Full recovery after 10 to 40 minutes of submersion can occur. CPR must be continued until the body has been warmed to at least 86° F (30° C). If still unresponsive at that temperature, the victim may be considered dead. It may take several hours of CPR while the patient is being properly rewarmed to make this determination.

The rewarming process for immersion victims should not be attempted in the field. The hospital management of victims of cold water submersion is very complex. They are best transferred to centers experienced with this problem, but they will never have a chance if rescuers do not implement CPR immediately.

FROST NIP

Frost nip, or very light frostbite, can be readily treated in the field if recognized early enough. This term is reserved for a form of superficial frostbite, but I am convinced that there really is a separate entity that should be considered as frost nip. The skin turns pure white in a small patch, generally the tip of the nose or ear edges. When detected, cup your hands and blow upon the affected parts to effect total rewarming. Under identical exposure conditions, some people are more prone to this than others. On one of my trips into sub-arctic Canada, a companion almost constantly frost nipped his nose at rather mild temperatures (20° F, 29° C). We frequently had to warn him, as he seemed oblivious to the fact that the tip of his nose would repeatedly frost.

FROSTBITE

Frostbite represents freezing of skin tissue. The temperature of the skin must be 24° F (4° C) before it will freeze. Risk for frostbite increases if the victim is hypothermic, dehydrated, injured, wearing tight fitting clothing or boots, or is not removing boots and changing socks or checking his feet at least nightly.

Traditionally, several degrees of frostbite are recognized, but the treatment for all is the same. The actual degree of severity will not be known until after the patient has been treated and the amount of damage then (readily) identified. In the wilderness, most cases of frostbite are not identified until the area has already thawed and the blue, discolored skin is found when finally changing socks or actually looking at the area in question.

When superficial frostbite is suspected, thaw immediately so that it does not become a more serious, deep frostbite. Warm the hands by withdrawing them into the parka through the sleeves—avoid opening the front of the parka to minimize heat loss. Feet should be thawed against a companion or cupped in your hands in a roomy sleeping bag or other insulated environment.

The specific therapy for a deep frozen extremity is rapid thawing in warm water (approximately 110° F, 43° C). This thawing may take 20 to 30 minutes, but it should be continued until all paleness of the tops of the fingers or toes has turned to pink or burgundy red, but no longer. This will be very painful and will require pain medication (Rx Lorcet 10/650 1 tablet, nasal Stadol, or injectable Nubain will probably be required).

Avoid opening the blisters that form. Do not cut skin away, but allow the digits to auto-amputate over the next 3 months. Blisters will usually last 2 to 3 weeks and must be treated with care to prevent infections (best done in a hospital with gloved attendants).

A black carapace will form in severe frostbite. This is actually a form of dry gangrene. This carapace will gradually fall off with amazingly good healing beneath. Efforts to hasten the carapace removal generally result in infection, delay in healing and increased loss of tissue. Leave these blackened areas alone. The black carapace separation can take over six months, but it is worth the wait. Without surgical interference, most frostbite wounds heal in six months to a year. All persons heading into the bush should already have had their tetanus booster (within the previous 10 years). Treat for shock with elevation of feet and lowering of the head, as this will frequently occur when these people enter a warm environment.

Once the victim has been thawed, very careful management of the thawed part is required. Refreezing will result in substantial tissue loss and this must be avoided. The patient sometimes becomes a stretcher case if the foot is involved, but not always. For that reason, it may be necessary to leave the foot or leg(s) frozen and allow the victim to walk back to the evacuation point or facility where the thawing will take place, realizing that the amount of damage is increasing the longer the area remains frozen. Early, rapid thawing is essential to minimize tissue loss. Do not allow the extremity to remain frozen unless it is essential to preserve life. Peter Freuchen, the great Greenland explorer, once walked days and miles keeping one leg frozen, knowing that when the leg thawed, he would be helpless. He lost his leg, but saved his life. And that's what will also happen to you. If you leave it frozen, you will lose the frozen part.

If a frozen member has thawed and the patient must be transported, use cotton between toes (or fluff sterile gauze from the emergency kit and place between toes) and cover other areas with a loose bandage to protect the skin during sleeping bag stretcher evacuation. The use of Spenco 2nd Skin for blister care would be ideal, see page 100. If a fracture also exits, immobilize when in the field, loosely so as not to impair the circulation any further.

PULMONARY CHILLING

Pulmonary chilling, sometimes called "frozen lung," occurs when breathing rapidly at very low temperatures, generally below -20° F (-29° C). There is burning pain, sometimes coughing of blood, frequently asthmatic wheezing and, with irritation of the diaphragm, pain in the shoulder(s) and upper stomach that may last for 1 to 2 weeks. The treatment is bed rest, steam inhalations, drinking extra water, humidification of the living area and no smoking. Avoid this condition by using parka hoods, face masks or breathing through mufflers which results in re-breathing the warmed, humidified, expired air.

IMMERSION FOOT

Immersion foot results from wet, cool conditions with temperature exposures from 68° F (20° C) down to freezing. This is an extremely serious injury that can be worse than frostbite. There are two stages of this problem: the first stage, in which the foot is cold, swollen, waxy, mottled with dark burgundy to blue splotches. This foot is resilient to palpation, whereas the frozen foot is very hard. Skin is sodden and friable. Loss of feeling makes walking difficult. The second stage lasts from days to weeks. The feet are swollen, red and hot; blisters form; infection and gangrene are common.

To prevent this problem, avoid non-breathing (rubber) footwear when possible, dry the feet and change wool socks when feet get wet or sweaty (every 3 to 4 hours, if necessary), periodically elevate, air, dry, massage the feet to promote circulation. Avoid tight, constricting clothing. As a minimum, remove boots and socks nightly, drying the feet and warming them before attempting to sleep.

Treatment differs from frostbite and hypothermia in the following ways: 1) Give the patient 10 grains of aspirin every 6 hours to help decrease platelet adhesion and clotting ability of the blood, 2) Give additional Lorcet 10/650 every 4 hours for pain, but discontinue as soon as possible, 3) Provide an ounce of hard liquor (30 ml) every hour while awake and 2 ounces (60 ml) every 2 hours during sleeping hours to vasodilate or increase the flow of blood to the feet. If you are unsure whether or not you are dealing with immersion foot or frostbite, or if you may have suffered both, treat as for frostbite.

CHILBLAINS

This results from exposure of dry skin to temperatures from 60° F (16° C) to freezing. The skin is red, swollen, frequently tender and itching. This is the mildest form of cold injury and no tissue loss results. Treatment is the prevention of further exposure with protective clothing over bare skin and the use of ointments if available, such as A & D Ointment or Vaseline (white petrolatum). The hydrocortisone 1% cream from the non-Rx kit Topical Bandaging Module will help when applied 4 times daily.

HEAT STRESS

High environmental temperatures are frequently aggravated by the amount of work being done, the humidity, reflection of heat from rock, sand or other structures (even snow!) and the lack of air movement. It takes a human approximately 10 days to become heat acclimated. Once heat stress adaptation takes place, there will be a decrease in the loss of salt in the sweat produced, thus conserving electrolytes. Another major change that occurs is the rapid production of sweat and the formation of larger quantities of sweat. Thus, the body is able to start its efficient cooling mechanism, sweating, more fully and with less electrolyte disturbance to the body.

Salt (NaCl) lost in sweat during work can normally be replaced at mealtime. An unacclimatized man working an 8 hour shift would sweat 4 to 6 liters of sweat. The salt content is high, namely 3 to 5 gram/liter of sweat. With acclimatization the salt concentration drops (1 to 2 gram/liter). Thus an acclimatized man might lose 6 to 16 grams of salt during an 8 hour shift in 6 to 8 liters of sweat. The unacclimatized man could lose a total of 18 to 30 grams of salt in 4 to 6 liters of sweat. The average American diet contains 10 to 15 grams/day of salt. This means that an unacclimatized worker could be in a 3 to 20 gram salt deficit per day. In the 10 days that it would take his body to become conditioned to heat stress, the total salt deficit could become substantial.

A concern in discussing heat illness preventions is the requirement that a heat stressed individual obtain adequate fluid replacement. If we focus on salt replacement, to the exclusion of adequate water intake, the individual may become salt loaded and accelerate his dehydration. Generally, however, an excess of salt or water over actual needs is readily controlled by kidney excretion.

However, depletion of body salt can lead to progressive dehydration because the body will attempt to maintain a balance between electrolyte concentration in tissue fluids with that in the cells. Deficient salt intake, with continued intake of water, tends to dilute tissue fluid. This suppresses antidiuretic hormone (ADH) of the pituitary gland, preventing the kidney from reabsorbing water. The kidney will then excrete a large volume of very dilute urine. The salt concentration of body fluids will be maintained, but at the cost of increasing the depletion of body water with a rapid onset of dehydration. Under heat stress, this can result in symptoms of heat exhaustion similar to those resulting from water restriction, but with more severe signs of circulatory insufficiency and notably little thirst. Absence of chloride in the urine (less than 3 gm/liter) is diagnostic of salt deficiency.

The ideal replacement fluid for the unacclimatized worker would be lightly salted water (0.1% or 1 tsp/gal), to prevent water or salt depletion. They will need 13 to 20 ounces of water before the activity and 3 to 6 ounces of water every 10 to 15 minutes during the active period. Water should not be withheld longer than 30 minute intervals. Replacement fluids should not contain greater sugar concentrations than 2.5 grams per 100 ml of water, as these higher concentrations slow gastric emptying. Acclimatized subjects will need only water as a replacement fluid, but will need 1 liter (32 ounces) per hour. Thirst may lag behind requirements, so that oral replacement should be voluntarily done before thirst even becomes noticeable. Water deprivation is dangerous and should be avoided.

With no water available, how long could a person expect to survive? The answer is generally dependent upon the temperature and the amount of activity. At a temperature of 120° F (49° C) with no water available, the victim would expect to survive about 2 days (regardless of activity). This temperature is so high that survival would not be increased beyond 2 days by even 4 quarts of water. Ten quarts might provide an extra day. At 90° F (32° C) with no water, the person could survive about 5 days if he walked during the day, 7 days if travel was only at night or if no travel was undertaken at all. With 4 quarts of water, survival would extend to 6.5 days with day travel and to 10 days with only night travel. With 10 quarts, days of survival would increase to 8 and 15 respectively. If the highest temperature was 60° (15.5° C) with no water, the active person could expect to survive 8 days, the inactive person 10 days.

HEAT CRAMPS

Salt depletion can result in nausea, twitching of muscle groups and at times severe cramping of abdominal muscles, legs, or elsewhere.

Treatment consists of stretching the muscles involved (avoid aggressive massage), resting in a cool environment, and replacing salt losses. Generally 10 to 15 grams of salt and generous water replacement should be adequate treatment.

HEAT EXHAUSTION

This is a classic example of compensatory shock (see page 16), but in this case encountered while working in a hot environment. The body has dilated the blood vessels in the skin to divert heat from the core to surface for cooling. However, this dilation is so pronounced, coupled with the profuse sweating and loss of fluid, also a part of the cooling process, that the blood pressure to the entire system falls too low to adequately supply the brain and the visceral organs. The patient will have a rapid heart rate, and will have the other findings associated with the compensatory stage of shock: pale color, nausea, dizziness, headache, and a light-headed feeling. Generally the patient is sweating profusely, but this may not be the case. The temperature may be elevated.

Treat as for shock. Have the patient lie down immediately, elevate the feet to increase the blood supply to the head, remove from direct sunlight and the hot environment. Provide copious amounts of water, a minimum of 1 to 2 quarts. Lightly salted water would be best. Obviously, fluids can only be administered if the patient is conscious. If unconscious, elevate the feet 3 feet above head level and protect from aspiration of vomit. Give water when the patient awakens.

HEAT STROKE (SUN STROKE)

Heat stroke represents the complete breakdown of the heat control process (thermal regulation) in the human body. There is generally a loss of the ability to sweat, core temperatures rise over 105° F (40° C) rapidly and will soon exceed 107.6° F (42° C) and result in death if this is not treated aggressively. THIS IS A TRUE EMERGENCY. It is a progressive stage of shock. The patient will be confused, very belligerent and uncooperative, and rapidly become unconscious. Immediately move into shade or erect a hasty barrier for shade. Spray with water or other suitable fluid and fan vigorously to lower the core temperature through evaporative cooling. This is the one time in medicine when it may be justifiable to piss on your patient. Massage limbs to allow the cooler blood of the extremities to return to core circulation more readily and fan to increase evaporative heat loss. Carefully monitor the core temperature and cease cooling when it lowers to 102° F (39° C). The temperature may continue to fall or suddenly raise again.

The most significant finding in heat stroke is the altered mental status of the victim. While heat exhaustion victims can be confused, this should resolve rapidly when they are in the shock treatment position (head down, feet up). The confusion and very often belligerent behavior of heat stroke victims make them very hard to handle. While their skin is normal dry and hot, this is not always the case. Suspect heat stroke in anyone who becomes confused and erratic in behavior, or unconscious, during exercise in a hot environment.

This person should be evacuated as soon as possible for his thermal regulation mechanism is quite unstable and will be labile for an undeterminable length of time. He should be placed under a physician's care as soon as possible. Terminate the expedition, if necessary, to evacuate.

PRICKLY HEAT

This is a heat rash caused by the entrapment of sweat in glands in the skin. This can result in irritation and frequently severe itching. Treatment includes cooling and drying the involved area and avoiding conditions that may induce sweating for awhile. Providing several hours of cool, dry environment daily is the only reliable treatment for prickly heat, but you may treat for itch as indicated on page 32.

LIGHTNING

Other than being totally toasted, cardiopulmonary arrest is the most significant lightning injury. People screaming from fright or burns after an electrical bolt has struck are already out of immediate danger. Their wounds may be dressed later. Those who appear dead must have immediate attention as they may be salvaged. Generally, when dealing with mass casualties the wounded are cared for preferentially, while the dead are left alone. Not in this instance! The victim is highly unlikely to die unless cardiopulmonary arrest happens. But if cardiopulmonary arrest does happen, 75% will die unless CPR is performed. As the heart tends to restart itself due to its inherent ability (automaticity), the heart beat may return spontaneously in a short time. The respiratory system, however, may be shut down for 5 to 6 hours before being able to resume its normal rhythm. The lack of oxygen this would cause will allow a person whose heart has started spontaneously to die. When administrating CPR, take precautions with the cervical spine for the force of the explosion associated with lightning may result in fractures of the neck or other portions of the body. While CPR is being performed, check for the pulse periodically. When the heart restarts, maintain ventilations for the patient until respirations also resume. Attempt to continue this as long as possible, for even after many hours the victim may revive with no neurological defects, but only if CPR or respiration ventilation has been properly performed. Remember, after a lightning strike the victim's eyes may be fixed and dilated, respirations ceased, heart stopped, blood pressure 0/0—all signs of clinical death. Pay no attention to these findings, but administer CPR as long as physically possible.

Lightning frequently causes vascular spasms in its victim. This can result in faint, or even non-palpable pulses. When the vasospasm clears, which it generally does within a few hours, the pulses return.

Neurological defects are the second major consequence of lightning hits. Approximately 72% of victims suffer loss of consciousness and three-quarters of these people will have a cardiopulmonary arrest. Direct damage to the brain can result, but frequently the neurological defects, to include seizure activity and abnormal brain wave studies, eventually revert to normal. Two thirds of victims will have neurological defects of the lower half of their bodies, one-third, paralysis of the upper half. Amnesia and confusion of events taking place after the accident are common, but usually transient.

Most will have amnesia, confusion, and short term memory loss that may last two to five days after the injury. These effects are similar to the electroconvulsive shock therapy used for certain psychiatric problems. The person may be able to talk intelligently, but shortly thereafter not remember the conversation had taken place—or even remember that they had ever seen the people they were talking to.

Burns from the lightning itself are generally not severe. Very high voltage is carried over the surface of conductors. The high voltage of lightning is similarly carried over the surface of the body with minimal internal burn damage, the so called "flashover effect."

Direct electrical burn damage can occur however, and when it does it usually consists of one of several types. Linear burns start at the head, progress down the chest, and split to continue down both legs. These burns are usually ½ to 1½ inches in width and are first and second degree. They follow areas of heavy sweat concentration. Punctate burns appear like a buck shot wound. These are full thickness third degree burns that are discrete, round wounds, measuring from a few millimeters to a centimeter in width. These seldom require grafting as the area is so small. Feathering or ferning burns are diagnostic of lightning injury. They fade within a few hours to days and require no treatment. This phenomena is not a true burn, but the effect of electron showers on the skin. They have a characteristic reddish fern appearance that covers the skin surface - particularly notable on the trunk. Thermal burns also result from vaporization of surface moisture, combustion of clothing, heated metal buckles, etc. Thermal burns are the most common type of lightning associated burn and they can be first, second, or third degree.

The flashover effect saves most victims from burn trauma. However, as noted, burns do occur. Persons with head burns are two and a half times more likely to die than those without. Possibly more surprising, persons with leg burns are five times more likely to die than those who do not have them. This is most likely related to a ground or step current phenomenon.

The four mechanisms of direct lightning injury are: 1) direct strike, 2) splash, 3) step current, 4) blunt trauma. To minimize the chance of lightning injury, the following should be noted about these mechanisms:

1). Direct strikes are most likely when in the open, especially if carrying metal or objects above shoulder level. Shelter should be taken within the cone of safety described as a 45° angle down from a tall object, such as a tree or cliff face.

2). Splash injuries are perhaps the most common mechanism of lightning hit—the current striking a tree or other object, may jump to a person whose body has less resistance than the object the lightning initially contacted. Splash injuries may occur from person to person, when several people are standing close together. It has jumped from fences after having struck the fence some distance away. It has splashed to people from plumbing fixtures inside houses that were struck. Avoid close proximity to walls, fences, plumbing, or other items that could be struck.

3). Step current is also called stride voltage and ground current. The lightning current spreads out in a wave along the ground from the struck object, with the current strength decreasing as the radius from the strike increases. If the victim's feet are at different distances from the point of the strike, and the resistance in the ground greater than through his body, he will complete a circuit. Large groups of people can be injured simultaneously in this manner. Keeping feet and legs together, while squatting down, minimizes the chances of step voltage injury.

4). Blunt trauma, or the sledgehammer effect, results from the force of the lightning strike, or the explosive shock wave which it produces. It may occur with the victim being forcibly knocked to the ground. Over 50% of victims will have their ear drums ruptured in one or both ears. This may result from direct thermal damage, the thunder shock wave, or even skull fractures from the blunt trauma. Barotrauma to the ears may be reduced by keeping the mouth open during times of great danger.

The above scenario has a person squatting with legs together and mouth open in a zone of safety, but not too near the nearby protective tree or cliff face. Spread party members out to maximize the chance that there will be survivors, and thus rescuers, if lightning strikes appear imminent. Get boats into a zone of safety near shore against the tree line or cliff face. Other than the immediate presence of lightning is there any warning? At times there will be the smell of ozone, hair may stand on end, and St Elmo's fire may be present. Good luck!

HIGH ALTITUDE ILLNESS

The high altitude related illnesses can generally be avoided by gradual exposure to higher elevation, with the camping or sleeping ascent rate not exceeding 1,000 feet (300 meters) per day when above 9,000 feet (2,800 meters). Alternatively, avoid sleeping at greater than 2,000 foot (600 meter) increments every 2 days when suddenly traveling from near sea level to 10,000 feet (3000 meters).

A high carbohydrate diet, consisting of at least 70 percent carbohydrates started 1 to 2 days prior to ascent, remaining well hydrated, and exercising moderately until altitude acclimatized, all help prevent high altitude illness.

The three major clinical manifestations of this disease complex are Acute Mountain Sickness (AMS), High Altitude Pulmonary Edema (HAPE), and High Altitude Cerebral Edema (HACE). As will be noted in the next three sections, the symptoms progress rather insidiously. They are not clear-cut, separate diseases—they often occur together. The essential therapy for each of them is recognition and descent. This is life saving and more valuable than the administration of oxygen or the drugs mentioned. To prevent them it is helpful to "climb high, but camp low"—ie, spend nights at the lowest camp elevation feasible.[17]

ACUTE MOUNTAIN SICKNESS (AMS)

Rarely encountered below 6,500 feet (2,000 meters), AMS is common in persons going above 10,000 feet (3,000 meters) without taking the time to acclimatize for altitude. Symptoms beginning soon after ascent consist of headache (often severe), nausea, vomiting, shortness of breath, weakness, and sleep disturbance.

A periodic breathing known to physicians as Cheyne-Stokes breathing may develop, but this does not necessarily lead to AMS.

Prevention, as with all of the high altitude illness problems, is gradual ascent beyond altitudes above 9,000 (2800 meters) feet and light physical activity for the first several days. For persons especially prone to AMS, it may be helpful to take acetazolamide (Diamox) prophylactically 125 mg every 12 hours starting the day of ascent and continuing the next 3 to 5 days. This medication helps prevent or treat the acid base imbalance of the blood which can occur in some people due to the increased loss of carbon dioxide at high altitudes. The treatment dose of acetazolamide is 250 mg twice daily for 5 days. This prescription drug should be added to your medical kit if you expect to encounter elevations above 9,000 feet. See further discussion of Diamox on page 213.

The best AMS treatment is descent and relief can often be felt even if the descent is only 2,000 to 3,000 feet (600 to 900 meters). Full relief can be obtained by descending to below 6,500 feet (2,000 meters). Stricken individuals should avoid heavy exercise, but sleep does not help as the breathing is slower during sleep and oxygen deprivation is worse. Oxygen will only help if taken continuously for 12 to 48 hours. Aspirin may be used for headache. Percogesic or ibuprofen from the Non-Rx Oral Medication Module may be used. In addition to descent, Decadron (dexamethasone) 4 mg tablets every 6 hours until below the altitude at which symptoms appeared has been shown to help control the symptoms of AMS. Decadron tablets or injection should be added to your medical kit if you expect to encounter elevations above 10,000 feet. See further discussion of decadron on pages 33 and 213.

HIGH ALTITUDE PULMONARY EDEMA (HAPE)

This problem is rare below 8,000 feet (2,500 meters), but occurs at higher altitude in those poorly acclimatized. It is more prone to occur in persons between the ages of 5 and 18 (the incidence is apparently less than .4% in persons over 21 and as high as 6% in those younger); in persons who have had this problem before; and in persons who have been altitude acclimatized and who are returning to high altitude after spending less than 2 weeks at sea level.

Prevention is altitude acclimatization as discussed in the section on AMS above. Taking nifedipine (Procardia) 20 mg every 8 hours during the ascent phase and for three additional days at altitude has been shown to work prophylactically (see page 196).

Symptoms develop slowly within 24 to 60 hours of arrival at high altitude with shortness of breath, irritating cough, weakness, rapid heart rate and headache which rapidly progress to intractable cough with bloody sputum, low-grade fever and increasing chest congestion. Symptoms may progress profoundly at night. Climbers should be evaluated by listening to their chests for a fine crackling sound (called rales) and resting pulse rate checked nightly. A pulse rate of greater than 110 per minute or respirations greater than 16 per minute after a 20 minute rest is an early sign of HAPE. Respirations over 20 per minute and pulse over 130 per minute indicates a medical emergency and the patient must be evacuated immediately. Without treatment, death usually occurs within 6 to 12 hours after onset of coma.

Descent to lower altitude is essential and should not be delayed. Treatment includes nifedipine 20 mg sublingual (or chewed and swallowed) given upon diagnosis and repeated every 6 hours. Oxygen may be of value if given continuously over the next 12 to 48 hours, starting at 6 liters/minute for the first 15 minutes, then reduced to 2 liters/minute. A snug face mask is better than nasal prongs. Oxygen may provide rapid relief in mild cases, however it should be continued for a minimum of 6 to 12 hours, if possible. Oxygen is not a substitute for descent in severe cases. A descent of as little as 2,000 to 3,000 feet (600 to 900 meters) may result in prompt improvement. The portable hyperbaric chamber called a Gamow

Bag is very useful in reversing the effects of high altitude (see Figure 31). When zippered shut with the patient inside, this nylon bag is pressurized with the use of a foot or mechanical pump. A difference of 2 pounds per square inch is formed when the bag is fully pressurized, resulting in a significant apparent decrease in altitude for the patient (see Table 9). Length of treatment time in the bag would be until symptoms cleared and the climbing conditions permit the aided descent of the patient.

FIGURE 31. *Gamow Bag used for simulating descent in the treatment of the high altitude illnesses.*

HIGH ALTITUDE CEREBRAL EDEMA (HACE)

HACE is a less common event than AMS or HAPE, but it is more dangerous. Death has occurred from HACE at altitude as low as 8,000 feet (2,500 meters), but HACE is rare below 11,500 feet (3,500 meters). The symptoms are increasingly severe headache, mental confusion, emotional behavior, hallucinations, unstable gait, loss of vision, loss of dexterity, and facial muscle paralysis. The victim may fall into a restless sleep, followed by a deep coma and death.

Descent is essential. The use of the Gamow Bag, as indicated above, can be life-saving. Oxygen should be administered starting at 6 liters/minute for the first 15 minutes, followed by a flow rate of 2 liters/minute. Decadron

TABLE 9

GAMOW BAG ALTITUDE REDUCTION TABLE

Simulated Descent

The following table shows the altitude that is simulated when using a Gamow Bag that is pressurized to 2 psi (103 mm Hg.) It can be seen that the maximum possible descent would be from the top of Everest at about 9000 m (29,529 ft) to about 6198 m (20,334 ft); **a descent of about 2800 m (9190 ft).**

Meters	Feet	mm Hg	Meters	Feet	mm Hg	▲Change (ft)
0	0	760	-1022	-3353	863	3353
300	984	731	-751	-2464	834	3448
600	1969	705	-495	-1624	808	3593
900	2953	679	-232	-761	782	3714
1200	3937	654	24	78	757	3859
1500	4921	630	288	945	733	3976
1800	5906	607	535	1755	710	4151
2100	6890	584	798	2618	687	4272
2400	7874	562	1054	3458	665	4416
2700	8859	541	1310	4298	645	4561
3000	9843	522	1555	5102	626	4741
3300	10827	503	1805	5922	607	4905
3600	11812	484	2053	6736	588	5076
3900	12796	466	2299	7543	570	5253
4200	13780	449	2544	8347	553	5433
4500	14765	433	2787	9144	537	5621
4800	15749	417	3028	9935	521	5814
5100	16733	401	3268	10722	505	6011
5400	17717	387	3505	11500	491	6217
5700	18702	372	3741	12274	476	6428
6000	19686	359	3975	13042	463	6644
6300	20670	345	4206	13800	449	6870
6600	21655	333	4436	14555	437	7100
6900	22639	320	4664	15303	424	7336
7200	23623	309	4890	16044	413	7579
7500	24608	297	5113	16776	401	7831
7800	25592	286	5335	17504	390	8088
8100	26576	276	5554	18223	380	8353
8400	27560	266	5771	18935	370	8625
8700	28545	256˙	5986	19640	360	8905
9000	29529	246	6198	20334	350	9195

(dexamethasone) should be given in large doses, namely 10 mg intra-venously, followed by 4 mg every 6 hours intramuscularly until the symp-toms subside. Response is usually noted within 12 to 24 hours and the dosage may be reduced after 2 to 4 days and gradually discontinued over a period of 5 to 7 days. Immediate descent and oxygen are recommended to prevent permanent neurological damage or death.

OTHER HIGH ALTITUDE CONDITIONS

Generalized swelling of the face, arms, and legs can appear after arrival at high altitude and may persist for days or even weeks. It is more common in women than men. The cause is unknown and no treatment is required. The swelling disappears after descent. The use of diuretics to eliminate this prob-lem should be discouraged as they can lead to increased problems with dehydration.

Hemorrhages of the retinal blood vessels (of the eye) can occur at altitude over 14,000 feet (4,300 meters) and is frequently found in climbers over 17,600 feet (5,365 meters). This condition rarely causes visual difficulty. There is no treatment. It resolves several weeks after return to sea level.

Increased flatulence may be noted in high altitude, a condition referred to in the medical journals as HAFE (High Altitude Flatulent Expulsion). Foods known to cause gas at lower altitude should be avoided. Simethicone products can be taken to help control this problem, such as Phazyme 125, 1 tablet with meals and at bed time. This medication is available without a prescription. A deluge of articles on this subject has caused several medical journals to decline publishing any further work on this topic. Actually, not much substance was contained in these articles.

High Altitude Cachexia (HAC) is the name that has been given to the extreme weight loss that climbers note on long high altitude climbs, above 17,000 feet (5,200 meters). Providing adequate amounts of carbohydrate seems to curtail some muscle loss. Fats and proteins become less palatable at high altitude. Climbers need between 5,000 and 6,000 kcal/day: 55% from carbohydrates, 35% from fats, and 10% from proteins.

Dehydration is a significant problem from respiratory loss in the cold, dry air and due to rapid breathing rates. Climbers become dehydrated, yet urinate a dilute urine, rather than concentrating and conserving body fluid as is usual under dehydration circumstances.

Vitamin intake should be approximately 3 times the recommended daily allowances due to the high calorie intake. To consume 6,000 kcal/day, a person would have to be in excellent physical shape. Most healthy young people cannot use more than 4,200 kcal/day, yet I have encountered wilderness brutes who required 8,000 kcal/day for weeks on end. Be sure that the cook's larder is ready for them or they can become very unhappy people.

Appendix A

THE WILDERNESS EXPEDITION MEDICAL KIT

Most injuries and conditions described in this book can be treated with very little in the way of kit components. But I have included here state-of-the-art items that would provide ideal treatment aid. As this book has been written for those who may be isolated without ready access to professional medical care, the treatments discussed go beyond normal first aid. The kit described in Appendix A similarly goes beyond what would be considered a "first aid" kit. But the initial modules are indeed easily useable under first aid conditions. The kit consists of 6 units: Topical Bandaging Module, Non-Rx Oral Medication Module, Orthopedic Module, Field Surgical Module, Rx Oral/Topical Medication Module, and the Rx Injectable Module.

As a minimum, the Topical Bandaging Module and Non-Rx Oral Medication Module will generally fulfill the vast majority of emergency treatment requirements. The Field Surgical Module and the prescription modules are designed for long term, and more advanced patient care. All items listed in the kit modules can be obtained without a prescription, except in the modules clearly marked "Rx."

All non-prescription medications have packaging that describes the official dosages and appropriate warnings or precautions concerning their use. Prescription medications have elaborate package inserts with this same information. When obtaining a prescription drug for your medical kit, request the package insert from your physician or copy the information for your use from the Physicians' Desk Reference (PDR), which is available at libraries and bookstores everywhere.

THE WILDERNESS EXPEDITION MEDICAL KIT
Topical Bandaging Module

Quantity	Item
2 pkgs	Coverstrip Closures ¼" x 3" (3/pkg)
1 pkg	Coverstrip Closures ½" x 4" (6/pkg)
6	Tegaderm 2⅜" x 2¾"
2	Spenco 2nd Skin 3" x 13"
2	Spenco Adhesive Knit Bandage 5" x 6"
15 pkg	Nu-Gauze, high absorbent, sterile, 2 ply, 3" x 3" (pkg/2)
3	Surgipad, Sterile, 8" x 10"
2	Elastomull, Sterile Roller Gauze, 4" x 162"
2	Elastomull, Sterile Roller Gauze, 2½" x 162"
25	Coverlet Bandage Strips 1" x 3"
1	Tape, Waterproof 1" x 5 yds
1	Hydrocortisone Cream 1%, 1 oz tube
1	Triple Antibiotic Ointment, 1 oz tube
1	Hibiclens Surgical Scrub, 4 oz bottle.
1	Dibucaine Ointment 1%, 1 oz tube
1	Tetrahydrozoline Ophthalmic Drops, .05%, 15 ml bottle
1	Starr Otic Drops, ½ oz bottle
1	Clotrimazole Cream, 2%, ½ oz tube
1 pair	Vinyl examination gloves
1	Over-pack Container for above

COVERSTRIP CLOSURES—by Beiersdorf is the best wound closure tape system that can be obtained. They can be removed and re-applied while trying to adjust the wound edges and still stick firmly—something that few tapes can do. These strips breathe and can be left on as long as necessary for the wound to heal, often without an outer covering. By far better than "butterfly" bandages, the latter can be substituted if cost and availability are factors.

TEGADERM—by 3M Corp. This is the "Gore-tex" of bandaging. This thin coating will seal water out, yet let a wound remain visible and breathe. It should be applied to wounds that are not seeping fluid or blood. They are ideal for covering cuts as the user can continue to immerse the wound in water while canoeing, working outside, etc, without contaminating the injury. Other similar products exist, but in my tests this brand sticks and breathes the best.

SPENCO 2ND SKIN—Truly a major advance in field medicine. This inert hydrogel consists of 96% water and 4% polyethylene oxide. It is used on wet, weeping wounds to absorb these fluids and protect the injury. This is a perfect prevention or cure for friction blisters. It revolutionized the field treatment of 1st, 2nd, and 3rd degree burns, as it can be applied to all three as a covering and for pain relief. This item should be in every medical kit. The ideal covering pad is the Spenco Adhesive Knit Bandage. If used in treating blisters, remove only the outer covering of cellophane from the 2nd Skin, cover with the Knit Bandaging, and occasionally dampen with clean water to maintain the hydrogel's hydration. It will last a lot longer that way when in short supply.

NU-GAUZE PADS—J&J Company has developed a gauze that is 2 ply yet it absorbs nearly 50% more fluid than conventional 12 ply gauze pads. This may not seem important until a rapidly bleeding wound needs care. For years J&J has made a "Nu-Gauze" strip packing dressing—the Nu-Gauze pads are a completely different material. They are a wonderful advance in gauze design.

SURGIPAD—An 8x10 sterile bandage for covering or compression of large wounds. This bandage can be used as a feminine sanitary napkin. If this large bandage is not carried, then several Kotex or equal should be carried in every trip medical kit.

ELASTOMULL ROLLER GAUZE—A superior rolled gauze by Beiersdorf, it stretches, does not unravel, and has low dust content. Its sterile packages are ideal for field use. The gauze can be applied directly over wounds, or used to hold other bandaging material in position.

COVERLET BANDAGE STRIPS—Another Beiersdorf product. These are common 1"x3" bandage strips, but they are the best made. They stick even when wet, will last through days of hard usage, and stretch for compression on a wound and conform for better application.

WATERPROOF TAPE—A tough tape that can be used for splinting or bandage application. There are no brand advantages that I can determine. A 1" by 5 yd roll on a metal spool is a useable size.

HYDROCORTISONE CREAM 1%—1 oz tube. This non-Rx steroid cream treats allergic skin rashes, such as those from poison ivy. A cream is ideal for treating weeping lesions, as opposed to dry scaly ones, but will work on either. To potentiate this medication apply an occlusive dressing (plastic cover) overnight.

TRIPLE ANTIBIOTIC OINTMENT—1 oz tube. Each gram of this ointment contains bacitracin 400 units, neomycin sulfate 5 mg and polymyxin B sulfate 5000 units. For use as a topical antibiotic in the prevention and treatment of minor infections of abrasions and burns. A light coat should be applied twice daily. Neomycin can cause skin rash and itch in some people. If this develops, discontinue use.

HIBICLENS SURGICAL SCRUB—This Stuart product [chlorhexidine gluconate 4%] far surpasses hexachlorophene and povidone-iodine scrub in its antiseptic action. Its onset and duration of action is much more impressive than either of those two products also.

DIBUCAINE OINTMENT 1%—1 oz tube. This is a topical anesthetic agent which will very effectively numb the skin for temporary relief of pain and itching associated with sunburn, minor burns, insect bites and stings, and hemorrhoids. Apply 3 or 4 times daily.

TETRAHYDROZOLINE OPHTHALMIC DROPS .05%—15 ml bottle. These eye drops are used for allergy relief and to remove red color and discomfort when due to smoke, eye strain, etc. It will not cure infection or cover the existence of a foreign body. Place 1 or 2 drops in each eye every 6 hours.

STARR OTIC DROPS—½ oz bottle. A formulation of chloroxlenol, benzalkonium chloride, acetic acid, and glycerine. More than 90% of all external otitis (outer ear infection, swimmer's ear) can be treated with acetic acid in a vehicle such as glycerine. A preparation may not be sold over the counter with an advertising claiming that it can cure ear infections, only for the purpose of softening wax and preventing infections. Use 3 drops 4 times a day, with a cotton plug.

CLOTRIMAZOLE CREAM 2%—½ oz tube. This is one of the most effective antifungal preparations available for foot, groin, or body fungal infections. Brand names are Lotrimin and Femestat (vaginal cream). The vaginal cream in a 2 ounce tube is less expensive per ounce and works well on the skin surface, as well as vaginally.

VINYL GLOVES—Due to concerns with hepatitis B and AIDS, it is prudent to carry vinyl gloves for first aid use. These can be non-sterile (they are readily sterilized by boiling or treating with antiseptics). Vinyl gloves will last much longer in a kit than latex gloves.

WILDERNESS EXPEDITION MEDICAL KIT
Non-Rx Oral Medical Module

Quantity	Item
24	Actifed Tablets (decongestant)
24	Percogesic Tablets (pain, fever, muscle spasm, sleep)
24	Ibuprofen 200 mg tab (pain, fever, inflammation)
24	Meclizine 25 mg tab (nausea, motion sickness prevention)
24	Benadryl 25 mg cap (antihistamine)
10	Bisacodyl 5 mg (constipation)
12	Imodium (diarrhea)
25	Mylanta (antacid)
6	1 oz Vials for repackaging the above
1	Over-pak Container for above

ACTIFED TABLETS—Decongestant. Each tablet contains 60 mg of pseudoephedrine (a vasoconstrictor that dries up mucus formation) and 2.5 mg of triprolidine (an antihistamine to block allergic reactions). Normal dose is 1 tablet every 6 hours to relieve congestion in nasal and sinus passages, and to treat pressure in the middle ear due to eustachian tube blockage. This item is available in generic products.

PERCOGESIC TABLETS—Relieves pain, fever, and muscle spasm. Each tablet contains 325 mg of acetaminophen and 30 mg of phenyltoloxamine citrate. Ideal for injuries of joints and muscles, as well as aches from infections. Phenyltoloxamine is also a decongestant, so that this product can replace the Actifed, but it is not quite as powerful. It also induces drowsiness and can be used as a sleeping aid and to calm a hysterical person. Dosage is generally 2 tablets every 4 hours as needed. One of the most useful non-Rx drugs obtainable.

IBUPROFEN TABLETS 200 MG—Relieves pain, fever, and inflammation. Overuse syndromes such as bursitis and tendinitis are common in wilderness related activities and this is an ideal treatment. The non-Rx dosage is 2 tablets, 4 times a day. Should be taken with food to prevent stomach irritation or heartburn. The Rx dosage is 4 tablets taken 4 times daily and this dose may be necessary for severe inflammation.

MECLIZINE TABLETS 25 MG—For nausea and vomiting, particularly when due to motion sickness. Dosage is 1 tablet daily. While sold non-Rx only for motion sickness, with prescription this may be taken 3 times daily for dizziness due to inner ear dysfunction. It will treat nausea from virtually any cause.

BENADRYL CAPSULES 25 MG—For antihistamine action, these capsules can be taken 1 or 2 every 6 hours. Benadryl is a powerful cough suppresser, the dose being 1 capsule every 6 hours.

BISACODYL 5 MG—A laxative that works on the large bowel to form a soft stool within 6 to 10 hours. Use 1 tablet as needed.

IMODIUM 2 MG—An anti-diarrheal with the generic name of loperamide. Dosage for persons 12 or older is 2 caplets after the first loose bowel movement followed by 1 caplet after each subsequent loose bowel movement, but no more than 4 caplets a day for no more than 2 days.

MYLANTA—High potency antacid tablets. Various brands may be substituted, but do not forget an antacid!

WILDERNESS EXPEDITION MEDICAL KIT
Orthopedic Module

Quantity	Item
1	Sam Splint
1	Elastic Bandage, 2"
1	Elastic Bandage, 3"
1	Elastic Bandage, 6"
1	Waterproof Tape, 1" x 5 yds

Quantity	Item
1	Unna Boot, 3" x 10 yds
2	Webril Orthopedic Padding, 3" x 4 yds
1	EMT Scissors
1	Over-pak Container for above

SAM SPLINT—A padded malleable splint that provides enough comfort to be used as a neck collar. It is adequately rigid to splint any extremity and universal so that only one of these need be carried for all splinting needs. This item replaces the necessity for ladder splints, etc. I have never recommended the inclusion of splints in wilderness medical kits, until this product was developed. It weighs less than 5 ounces.

ELASTIC BANDAGE, 2 inch

ELASTIC BANDAGE, 3 inch

ELASTIC BANDAGE, 6 inch

Obtain good quality bandages that stretch without narrowing and which provide firm, consistent support.

WATERPROOF TAPE, 1" x 5 YDS

UNNA BOOT—Casting material. This unusual item is of great assistance in treating sprains of the ankle, but can form supportive bandaging in many areas. It is a gauze strip coated with glycerine, gum arabic, zinc oxide, boric acid, and castor oil. When over-wrapped with an elastic bandage, it forms a durable, almost cast-like, supportive protection that can be easily removed by unwrapping or cutting with scissors. The best size is 3" by 10 yards. The sticky coating easily washes off your hands after wrapping and it serves to protect the skin of the wrapped body part. May be left on for 10 days if necessary.

WEBRIL ORTHOPEDIC PADDING—3" x 4 YDS. Long strand cotton fiber padding that provides excellent cushioning for splints of all types. I use it frequently to provide a wrap next to the skin, which can then be covered with an elastic (Ace) bandage for a secure, supportive soft cast.

EMT SCISSORS—Serrated shears that cut through clothing, sheet metal, bandaging, etc.

WILDERNESS EXPEDITION MEDICAL KIT
Non-Rx Field Surgical Module

Quantity	Item
3	3-0 Nylon Sutures
3	5-0 Nylon Sutures
1	3-0 Gut Suture
1	Needle Holder
1	Curved Hemostats
1	Straight Hemostats
1	Operating Scissors
1	Iris Scissors
1	Bandage Scissors, Lister
1	#3 Stainless Steel Scalpel Handle
3	#11 Scalpel Blades
3	#10 Scalpel Blades
1	Splinter Forceps
1	Adson Tissue Forceps with Teeth
15 pkg	Nu-Gauze, high absorbent, sterile, 2 ply, 3" x 3" (pkg/2)
1	Bulb Irrigating Syringe
2	Elastomull, Sterile Roller Gauze, 4" x 162"
2	Elastomull, Sterile Roller Gauze, 2½" x 162"
1	Tape, Waterproof 1" x 5 yds
2	Surgical Scrub Brushes, Povidone-Iodine
10 pkg	Q-Tips, Sterile (2/pkg)
1	Over-pak Container for above

SUTURE, NYLON 3-0

SUTURE, NYLON 5-0

SUTURE, PLAIN GUT 3-0—For use in repairing wounds, see page 91 in the text. Nylon sutures are 18 inches long with a curved needle attached. The plain gut suture is 27 inches long, packed in isopropyl alcohol. All packages are sterile.

NEEDLE HOLDER—The Mayo-Hegar needle holder, or equal, is necessary to hold the curved suture needle. See text, page 209, for information about its use.

FIGURE 32. *Mayo-Hegar Needle Holder.*

HEMOSTATS, CURVED AND STRAIGHT—These instruments are handy for fine work, such as tagging the ends of suture before tying, suture removal, clamping spurting vessels, and many other gory details. They are useful in disrupting loculations in abscess cavities. Hemostats look much like needle holders, but have shorter handles and are lighter in weight.

OPERATING SCISSORS—Sharp pointed scissors designed to cut through macerated tissue, sutures, and other surgical work.

IRIS SCISSORS—Very delicate, for removing small slivers of skin, aiding in removing foreign bodies, cutting tiny sutures, etc. Basically, these are a petite version of operating scissors.

BANDAGE SCISSORS, LISTER—Bandage scissors have been designed to protect the patient with one blunt end and the other end not only blunt, but with a smooth, snag free knob to allow easy sliding under a tight bandage.

FIGURE 33. *Operating and Lister Bandage Scissors.*

SCALPEL HANDLE, #11 AND #10 BLADES—Used for a variety of purposes, such as opening an abscess. The blades are sterile and individually sealed in protective packaging. The handle must be sterilized with boiling water, alcohol, etc., before use. The blades are disposable and snap onto the handle. I use a needle holder when snapping them off!

FIGURE 34. *Scalpel Handle, with a #11 blade and a #10 blade.*

SPLINTER FORCEPS—A fine pointed tweezer, for removal of foreign bodies.

ADSON TISSUE FORCEPS WITH TEETH—One side has one tooth, the other two teeth that interlock together for a slip-proof grasp of delicate tissue. Use to hold wound edges together for proper placement of butterfly bandages, tape strips, sutures, or even skin staples.

FIGURE 35. *Adson Tissue Forceps.*

BULB IRRIGATING SYRINGE—Jets water into a wound with considerable force to remove residue that will promote infection (see Figure 8, page 87).

WILDERNESS EXPEDITION MEDICAL KIT
Rx Oral/Topical Medication Module

Quantity	Item
20	Doxycycline 100 mg tablets (antibiotic)
20	Cefzil 250 mg tablets (antibiotic)
16	Floxin 400 mg tablets (antibiotic)
24	Lorcet 10/650 tablets (pain, cough)
24	Atarax 25 mg tablets (nausea, antihistamine, pain medication augmentation)
1	Topicort .25% Ointment, $^1/_2$ oz tube (skin allergy)
1	Neosporin Ophthalmic Ointment, $^1/_8$ oz tube (eye, ear antibiotic)
1	Tetracaine Ophthalmic Solution .5%, $^1/_8$ oz tube (eye, ear anethetic)
1	Kenalog in Orabase, 5 gm tube (mouth sores)
1	Stadol, Nasal Spray (pain)
*	Diamox 250 mg tablets, 10 per person (acute mountain sickness prevention and treatment)
*	Procardia 20 mg capsules (12 per climber at high risk—high altitiude pulmonary edema)
*	Decadron 4 mg tablets (10 per trip—allergy) (16 per climber at high risk—acute mountain sickness)
*	Chloroquine, 300 mg base. (malaria prevention) taken once weekly, beginning 1 week before leaving home and continued for 6 weeks after leaving malarious area. See text, page 171.
*	Larium (mefloquin) 250 mg. (malaria protection)

DOXYCYCLINE—The generic name of an antibiotic that is useful in treating many travel related diseases. The various sections of the text dealing with infections will indicate the proper dosage, normally 1 tablet twice daily. Not to be used in children eight years or younger or during pregnancy. May cause skin sensitivity on exposure to sunlight, thus causing an exaggerated sunburn. This does not usually happen, but be cautious during your first sun exposure when on this product. Many people traveling in the tropics have used this antibiotic safely. Like any oral medication this product may also cause allergic reactions. Very useful in malaria prevention at a dose of 1 tablet daily. Common brand names are Vibramycin, Vibra-tabs, Vivox, and Doryx.

CEFZIL 250 MG—A third generation cephalosporin antibiotic, this is very useful in treating sore throats, upper respiratory infections, pneumonias, soft tissue infections, and some causes of diarrhea. About 10% of people allergic to penicillin might be allergic to this drug.

FLOXIN 400 MG—A broad spectrum antibiotic of a group known as fluoroquinolones. This medication is useful in treating resistant organisms to the above antibiotics and diarrhea. Avoid excessive sun exposure while on this medication. Avoid in persons under the age of 18 and during nursing and pregnancy. Drink extra water when on this medication. Do not take with antacid, vitamins containing minerals, ibuprofen, or at meal times.

LORCET 10/650—The brand name of the combination of 650 mg of acetaminophen and 10 mg of hydrocodone, the principle use of the drug is in the relief of pain. Hydrocodone is a powerful cough suppressor. Also useful in treating abdominal cramping. The dosage of 1 tablet every 6 hours will normally control a severe toothache. Maximum dosage is 6 tablets per day. It may be augmented with Atarax—see below.

STADOL, NASAL INHALED—This powerful pain medication is formulated to be absorbed by the nasal mucosa. It is ten times stronger than morphine on a milligram to milligram basis. Use only one spray up a nostril and wait, the instructions say 60 to 90 minutes before using a second spray in the other nostril. This process may be repeated in 3 to 4 hours. It should be working effectively within 20 minutes, however, after the first spray. Overspraying and allowing the medication to drain down the throat will waste it since it is inactivated by gastric fluids.

ATARAX 25 MG—A brand name of hydroxyzine hydrochloride (note also the listing under "Vistaril" in the Rx Injectable Medication Module). These tablets have multiple uses. They are a very powerful anti-nausea agent, muscle relaxant, antihistamine, anti-anxiety agent, sleeping pill, and narcotic potentiator. For sleep 50 mg at bed time; for nausea 25 mg every 4 to 6 hours; to potentiate a narcotic, take a 25 mg tablet with each dose of the pain medication. This medication helps with rashes of all types and has a drying effect on congestion. The injectable version, Vistaril, has identical actions.

TOPICORT OINTMENT .25%—This Rx steroid ointment treats severe allergic skin rashes. Dosage is a thin coat twice daily. Occlusive dressings are not required when using this product. Should be used with caution over large body surface areas or in children. Use should be limited to 10 days or less, particularly in the latter cases.

NEOSPORIN OPHTHALMIC OINTMENT—⅛ oz tube. Same contents of "triple antibiotic ointment" listed above. Designed for use in the eye—can be melted into the ear. Can be instilled in either location 2 to 3 times daily for infection. Allow to melt.

TETRACAINE OPHTHALMIC SOLUTION (Drops)—15 ml bottle. Sterile solution for use in eye or ear to numb pain. Do not reapply to eye if pain returns without examining for foreign body very carefully. Apply periodically as needed for eye pain. Do not use in ears if considerable drainage is present for an ear drum may have ruptured. Avoid use if the ear drum is ruptured as this solution will cause profound vertigo (dizziness).

KENALOG IN ORABASE—5 gm tube. For use on mouth sores. May be applied every 3 hours, but generally 3 times daily is sufficient. This medication also works on the skin surface to treat localized itchy areas. See discussion, page 55.

DIAMOX—The brand name of acetazolamide. Used in the prevention of acute mountain sickness for those contemplating rapid ascent to elevations over 9,000 feet. Side effects include tingling of the mouth and fingers, numbness, loss of appetite, and occasional instances of drowsiness and confusion—almost all signs of the acute mountain sickness that one is trying to prevent. Increased urination and rare sun sensitive skin rash is encountered. See text, page 195.

DECADRON 4 MG—For allergy ½ tablet twice daily after meals for 5 days. For treatment of acute mountain sickness give 8 mg initially, then 4 mg every 6 hours until well below altitude at which symptoms appeared. See text, pages 33, 196, and 199.

CHLOROQUINE OR MEFLOQUINE—Used to prevent malaria. See text, page 171.

WILDERNESS EXPEDITION MEDICAL KIT
Rx Injectable Medication Module

Quantity	Item
1	Nubain 20 mg/ml, 10 ml multi-use vial (pain)
1	Lidocaine 1% 10 ml multi-use vial (local anesthetic)
12	3½ ml syringes with 25 gauge, ⅝ inch needles
1+	Decadron 4 mg/ml, 5 ml multi-use vial (steroid) 1 per trip for allergy; 3 vials per climber at risk for acute mountain sickness
10–15	Rocephin, 500 gm vials (antibiotic)
1	Vistaril 50 mg/ml, 10 ml multi-use vial (many uses)
1–2	Anakit or Anaguard (bee stings—anaphylactic shock, asthma)

NUBAIN 20 MG/ML—Strong, synthetic narcotic analgesic, it is available only by prescription, but it is not a controlled narcotic with the increased legal problems associated with those substances. Normal adult dose is 10 mg (½ ml) given intramuscularly every 3 to 6 hours. Can be mixed with 25 to 50 mg of Vistaril in the same syringe for increased analgesia in severe pain problems. It comes in 10 ml multi-use vials.

LIDOCAINE 1%—Injection for numbing wounds. Maximum amount to be used in a wound in an adult should be 15 ml. This fluid is also used to mix the Rocephin. See text, page 215 and package insert which comes with the Rocephin.

SYRINGES—Many types are available, but for wilderness use I find the 3½ ml with the attached 25 gauge, 5/8 inch needle to be the most universal. The best brand is Monoject as each syringe with needle is packed in a tough, sterile plastic case.

DECADRON 4 MG/ML—For use in allergic reactions, give 4 mg daily for 5 days IM. For Acute Mountain Sickness give 8 mg (2 ml) IM initially, then 4 mg (1 ml) every 6 hours until well below the altitude where symptoms started. High Altitude Cerebral Edema (HACE) requires larger doses. See pages 195 and 197.

ROCEPHIN 500 MG VIALS—A broad spectrum antibiotic of the cephalosporin class, the injectable medication has a wide range of bactericidal activities. Each vial will require 1.8 ml of lidocaine 1% to mix the contents. The reconstituted medication is stable at room temperatures for 3 days.

VISTARIL 50MG/ML—A brand name of hydroxyzine hydrochloride (note also the listing under "Atarax" in the Rx Oral Medication Module). Uses and dosages are the same as indicated in that listing. Obviously in the treatment of profound vomiting, injections of medication will work better than oral administration. This solution can be mixed in the same syringe as the Nubain for administration as one injection.

ANAKIT—A commercial kit consisting of a multiple use syringe of epinephrine (Adrenalin) and chewable antihistamine tablets, with alcohol wipes and bandage. One half the syringe amount (.3 ml) can be given before a twist is required to administer the second half of the injection. 0.3 ml is the standard adult dose required to treat anaphylactic shock due to severe allergic reactions from bee stings, etc. The Anaguard consists of the multiple injection syringe only. As with the syringe in the Anakit, it is to be used only on one person. See page 146 in text.

Appendix B

ADULT IMMUNIZATIONS AND DOSAGE SCHEDULES

This section has been designed particularly for the adventure traveler. Providing adequate time for proper pre-trip medical travel consultation and immunization cannot be stressed too strongly. Not only must vaccine administration be sequenced properly, but one requires a recovery time from possible reactions and time to acquire personal and prophylactic medications.

Prior to any trip out of the country, call the U.S. Department of State Advisory Hotline at (202) 647-5225 for the latest information concerning political unrest. This number includes health issues at times. Also call the Centers for Disease Control and Prevention International Travelers' Hotline at (404) 332-4559.[18] Contact IAMAT (The International Association For Medical Assistance to Travellers) for their latest immunization recommendations and membership packet. Membership is free, but a donation is appreciated. In the U.S. their address is: 417 Center Street, Lewiston, NY 14092 (716) 754-4883; in Canada: 40 Regal Road, Guelph, Ontario, N1K 1B5 (519) 836-0102.

CHOLERA

Primary immunization consists of two doses given subcutaneously or intramuscularly 1 week to 1 month or more apart. Booster injections are required every 6 months. Dosages are: children 6 months to 5 years, 0.2ml; 5 to 10 years, 0.3 ml; over 10 years, 0.5 ml. This immunization only provides approximately 30% to 50% protection. Immunization is effective 6 days after receiving an injection, immediately, if it was a booster. The International Certificate of Immunization must be validated with the use of a Uniform Stamp (see above) and will not be considered valid for 6 days from the time of immunization. This vaccine is generally not recommended for use in travelers due to its low level of effectiveness. If it is to be taken, a new dosage regimen of 0.1 ml given intradermally causes less side effects and still fulfills potential requirements for this vaccination that some government officials might demand. No government officially requires this vaccine, but some border crossing guards demand certification that you have had this vaccine. This problem is limited to a few African countries at this time. Side effects include: pain at the injection site for 24-48 hrs; possible local redness and swelling; fever, headache, malaise developing in most recipients and persisting for 1-2 days.

HEPATITIS A (INFECTIOUS HEPATITIS)

A single dose of pooled immune globulin (10% solution) protects against or modifies this form of hepatitis which is commonly caught from tainted food or water supplies. It must not be given at the same time as the Measles, Mumps, Rubella (MMR) vaccine. It may be given at least 14 days after MMR or 6 weeks to 3 months (preferably 6 months) before MMR. There are no apparent problems in the administration of Oral Polio Vaccine or Yellow Fever vaccine with or near immune globulin administration. Dosage depends upon body weight and length of time of required protection. At maximal doses it still must be repeated every 6 months for continued protection. If the traveler finds himself still overseas after six months, it is best to avoid receiving booster doses from questionable sources, but rather to take one's chances with possibly contracting Hepatitis A. It is better to contend with a miserable, yet very seldom serious disease such as Hepatitis A, than to risk acquiring more serious diseases such as Hepatitis B or AIDS from contaminated local supplies. Travelers making frequent foreign journeys to areas at risk for Hepatitis A should consider having their Hepatitis A IgG levels measured, as the presence of natural antibodies would indicate lifelong immunity without need for booster shots of immune globulin. Side effects are minimal other than rather mild possible pain at the injection site. This injection must be given in the gluteal muscles. A new vaccine that will provide longterm active immunity against Hepatitis A is available in Europe. Licensure is expected in the United States in mid-1994.

TABLE 10		
IMMUNE GLOBULIN DOSAGE*		
weight	short term(< 3 months)	long term (>3 months)
< 50 pounds	0.5 ml	1.0 ml
50-100 pounds	1.0 ml	2.5 ml
> 100 pounds	2.0 ml	5.0 ml
(repeat every 6 mos.)		
*Also called immune serum globulin and gamma globulin.		

HEPATITIS B (SERUM HEPATITIS)

This disease is most commonly spread by hypodermic usage, sexual contact, and blood transfusions. It has a very high prevalence in many areas of the world. Immunization is from a series of 1.0 ml IM injections of Hepatitis B Vaccine (Recombinant), called "Recombivax HB" by the manufacturer, Merck & Company. It is given on day 0, 1 month, and 6 months. Wholesale cost as of May 1994 is about $135.00 for 1 full course of immunization. Duration of protection and need for revaccination has not been defined. A blood test to determine adequate antibody response can be performed. If the antibody level falls below 10 SRUs, revaccination with 1.0 ml of vaccine should be considered. The injection must be given in the deltoid muscle. Side effects include: pain, inflammation at injection site; fatigue/weakness and low grade temp; nausea and diarrhea; sore throat and upper respiratory symptoms in 1% or slightly greater of recipients.

JAPANESE ENCEPHALITIS

Immunization requires 3 doses to be given at weekly intervals, with a booster dose at 12 to 18 months and at 4 year intervals thereafter, if risk continues. This vaccine is now available in the U.S. Reactions are infrequent. There have been no reports of demyelinating disease or encephalitis from the vaccine. Fever and local reactions develop in fewer than 10% of recipients. This vaccine should not be taken by pregnant women and persons with malignant diseases or other current illness.

INFLUENZA

Vaccines are prepared that give 1 to 2 years of immunity for prevalent strains of influenza A or B. New strains are constantly arising that require formulation of new vaccines to compensate for this "antigenic drift." Dosage is 0.5 ml IM in the deltoid muscle, given in the fall of the year. This vaccine is not required for routine travel, but may be suggested for the traveler heading into an epidemic area. Being confined on airplanes for long flights places you at high risk as the air breathed by everyone on the plane is recirculated. A booster of 0.5 ml must be given yearly. Fewer than 1/3 of recipients have local soreness around the injection for less than 2 days; fever, muscle ache, malaise can begin 6-12 hours after injection and last 1 or 2 days; persons with very severe egg allergy have increased risk of allergic reaction.

MEASLES, MUMPS, RUBELLA

One 0.5 ml dose given subcutaneously provides initial immunity. The MMR vaccine provides adequate protection against all three viral diseases, but each vaccine is available separately. The vaccine may not be given if the person is allergic to eggs or neomycin without special desensitization. This vaccine must be given at least 14 days prior to or 6 weeks to 3 months after immune serum globulin. While no booster shots are suggested routinely for mumps and rubella, all persons born after 1956 should receive a booster of measles containing vaccine to be considered immune. Side effects for these vaccines are as follows. Measles: low grade fever (99° to 102° F; 37° to 39°C) may occur 5-12 days after injection, rarely a generalized rash develops; fever higher than 103° F (39.4° C) occurs less than 15% of the time. Allergy to chicken eggs and neomycin may cause an allergic reaction. Mumps: burning and stinging of short duration at injection site; occasional mild fever; fever above 103° F is uncommon; allergic reactions at the injection site are extremely rare; swelling of the parotid salivary gland—low incidence; testicle inflammation is very rare; seizures, deafness, and encephalitis are very rare. Allergy to chicken eggs or feathers or to neomycin may cause an allergic reaction. Any active infection is reason to delay receiving this vaccine. Also, any blood disorders, immune deficiency or use of corticosteroid is a contraindication for vaccination. Rubella: Occasional moderate fever (101° to 102° F) less commonly high fever (over 103° F) burning at injection site; reactions are usually mild and transient, but include fever, rash, sore throat, nausea, vomiting, and joint ache. Avoid giving during pregnancy, to persons with blood disorders, or to those receiving corticosteroid. Allergy to neomycin may cause an allergic reaction. Avoid giving if active illness is present.

MENINGOCOCCAL MENINGITIS

This vaccine need be used only under special circumstances (military personnel in the U.S. and persons traveling to areas of the world where meningococcal infection is epidemic). The A/C/Y/W135 vaccine by Squibb-Connaught is given 0.5 ml subcutaneously. Duration of protection is unknown, but appears to be at least 3 years in those over 4 years of age. A booster shot of 0.5 ml must be given every 3 years. There might be local redness at injection site for 1-2 days. Reactions are uncommon and usually mild.

PLAGUE

In most countries of Africa, Asia and the Americas where plague is reported, the risk of exposure exists primarily in rural mountainous or upland areas. Adult immunization consists of 3 injections of 0.5 ml, 0.5 ml, and 0.2 ml (in that order) about 4 weeks apart and two boosters of 0.2 ml 6 months apart, then one dose every 1 to 2 years if needed. Side Effect Profile: Local pain and inflammation is the most common side effect; generalized fever and illness is uncommon.

PNEUMONIA

A vaccine against streptococcal (formerly called pneumococcal) pneumonia has been developed for high risk patients with chronic diseases or respiratory problems. One 0.5 ml IM injection in the deltoid muscle probably provides a life-long immunity. No booster immunization required. Side Effect Profile: Local inflammation and pain at the injection site is relatively common.

POLIOMYELITIS

Trivalent oral polio vaccine (OPV) is the vaccine of choice for all infants, children, and adolescents (up to their 18th birthday). The primary series is 3 doses, with dose 2 given at least 6 weeks after 1 and dose 3 given 8-12 months after dose 2. A supplemental dose is given to children at age 4 to 6 years. Anyone having a partial series may continue with the next dose(s), regardless of how long before the last dose was given. Unimmunized adults should be given the four full dose series of injectable inactivated polio vaccine (IPV)(3 doses given at 1 to 2 month intervals, followed by a 4th dose 6 to 12 months after the 3rd dose), if time allows, or a minimum of 2 doses of IPV given a month apart. If less than a month remains prior to departure, the administration of a single dose of OPV may be justified in case of potential high risk of exposure to wild poliovirus and the more rapid protective effect of OPV.

The good news is that there has been a significant decrease in wild strains of polio in the past few years, due to the massive world immunization program. There are very slight chances of adverse reactions with either polio vaccine. Vaccine associate disease is 1 per (oral) 8.7 million doses; disease in contacts incidence is 1 per 5.1 million doses. Any active infection is reason to delay receiving this vaccine. Also any blood disorders, immune deficiency or use of corticosteroid is a contraindication for vaccination. No vaccine associated disease reported with the injectable vaccine. There is a slight chance of allergy in people sensitive to cow serum, neomycin, and streptomycin.

RABIES

A pre-exposure regimen of rabies vaccine is appropriate for persons routinely exposed to potential rabid animals - including skunks, fox, raccoon and bats. It does not eliminate the need for additional therapy after rabies exposure, but simplifies post-exposure therapy by eliminating the requirement for rabies immune globulin (RIG) and by decreasing the number of doses of vaccine required. Prevention with human diploid cell vaccine (HDCV) is 3 doses given 1.0 ml IM in the deltoid muscle on days 0, 7, and 21 or 28. A new dosage of 0.1 ml intradermally given on the same dosage schedule also seems effective for prophylaxis. Caution should be taken to avoid taking chloroquine for malaria prophylaxis while receiving rabies immunization as it has been shown to reduce the antibody response.

Post-exposure immunization for those previously immunized is 2 doses (1 ml each) on days 0 and 3, with no RIG. If no prior immunization, give RIG 20 IU/kg (½ in bite site and ½ IM) and 5 doses (1 ml each) of HDCV on days 0, 3, 7, 14, and 28. These injections must be given in the deltoid muscle as two incidents of failure of post-exposure immunization with RIG and HDCV have occurred when these injections were given in the gluteal muscle.

To determine if a booster is needed, obtain antibody testing every two years. There is a very low incidence of side effect with the new diploid cell vaccine; some local irritation possible and occasional muscle ache and headache. In persons receiving a booster shot up to 6% may have hives, lymph node enlargement, and fever.

TETANUS - DIPHTHERIA

All persons should have a tetanus booster every 10 years; 5 years for puncture wounds, bites, and other contaminated wounds. This vaccine is so effective, that a booster sooner than every 10 years is probably not required. Dosage is 0.5 ml of dT vaccine given IM. A different vaccine is prepared for use in children. Infants receive a special diphtheria-tetanus-pertussis vaccine which is also a different formulation than that used in children. Family physicians, pediatricians, and travel medicine clinics generally have all three vaccines in stock at all times. Both adult and children's vaccines should be given with diphtheria toxoid in combination. Infants should follow the routine pediatric immunization schedule with the tetanus-diphtheria-pertussis-Hib combination vaccine. A local reaction at injection site is possible; fever may occur; severe allergic reactions are rare.

TYPHOID

Immunization should be completed before heading into areas where typhoid fever is known to be epidemic (many countries of Africa, Asia, and Central and South America). The vaccine is from 70% to 90% effective in preventing the disease and also decreases the severity of the disease. Immunization consists of two 0.5 ml doses given 1 month apart, with a booster dose every 3 years. An intradermal dose of 0.1 ml may be substituted after the initial 0.5 ml dose has been received. A new high potency oral vaccine became available in 1990 which provides at least 80% effective protection and which has considerably less side effects than the current vaccine. Immunization is with one capsule of the live attenuated Ty21a (Vivotif) vaccine, taken every other day for four doses (day 0, 2, 4, 6). Booster requirement for the injectable vaccine is 0.5 ml subcutaneously (or 0.1 ml intradermal) every 3 years. Local pain at the injection site occurs in most recipients; fever, lethargy, headache may last for 1-2 days. Safe for use when pregnant. Allergy to phenol may cause an allergic reaction. Booster requirement for the oral vaccine has not been determined. The current recommendation is that the full four capsule treatment dose be repeated every five years.

YELLOW FEVER

Immunization is required for travel to many countries in South America, Africa and Asia. The immunization consists of one 0.5 ml injection, which confers immunity for 10 years. It is available only at designated Yellow Fever Vaccination Centers (check your County or State Board of Health for the nearest facility). The booster dose is the same amount every 10 years. Approximately 5% to 10% of recipients have headache, lethargy, muscle ache and fever which occurs 5-10 days after vaccination.

SCHEDULE PRIOR TO DEPARTURE

Taking into account the incompatibility of some vaccines, the number of doses required to effectively complete some series, and the delay until some immunizations are considered valid, an immunization schedule has to be established starting approximately 8 weeks prior to departure.

A sample immunization schedule for someone requiring various series of live and killed vaccines is diagrammed below. This schematic also indicates the start of malaria prophylaxis with chloroquine or mefloquine.

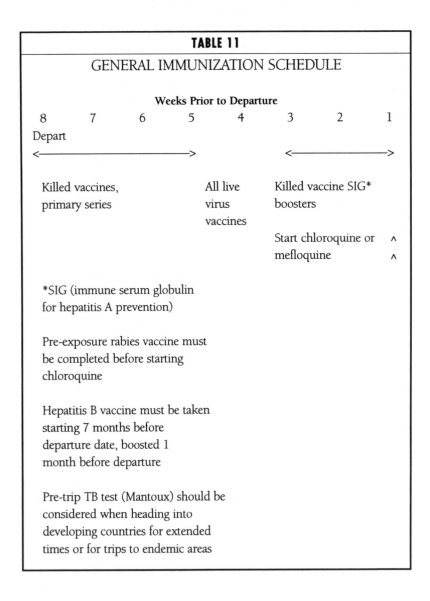

TABLE 11

GENERAL IMMUNIZATION SCHEDULE

Weeks Prior to Departure

8	7	6	5	4	3	2	1

Depart

<────────────────────>   <────────────>

Killed vaccines,   All live   Killed vaccine SIG*
primary series   virus   boosters
                                  vaccines

                                                      Start chloroquine or   ∧
                                                      mefloquine   ∧

*SIG (immune serum globulin
for hepatitis A prevention)

Pre-exposure rabies vaccine must
be completed before starting
chloroquine

Hepatitis B vaccine must be taken
starting 7 months before
departure date, boosted 1
month before departure

Pre-trip TB test (Mantoux) should be
considered when heading into
developing countries for extended
times or for trips to endemic areas

Appendix C

SUGGESTED READINGS AND REFERENCES

Auerbach, Paul S. Medicine for the Outdoors, 2nd Ed 1991, 347 pages. Little, Brown, and Company, Waltham MA

A founder and past president of the Wilderness Medical Society, Dr Auerbach presents a knowledgeable overview of the entire wilderness medical field. This text is patterned after his large text of wilderness medicine, but written for the lay reader.

Bonney, Bruce F. and Jack K. Drury. The Backcountry Classroom, 1992, 288 pages. ICS Books, Merrillville, IN

This book contains the lesson plans of the Wilderness Education Association for teaching various wilderness related activities. From skills as basic as cooking to complex issues such as judgement and decision making.

Bowman, Warren D. Outdoor Emergency Care, 1988, 466 pages. National Ski Patrol, Lakewood, CO

This book is one of the best sources of information on the medical aspects of cold and snowy camping, orthopedic injuries, and dealing with multiple casualties.

Cockrell, David Ed. The Wilderness Educator, 1991, 194 pages. ICS Books, Merrillville, IN

A college level text describing the curriculum of the Wilderness Education Association which stresses an understanding of group dynamics, leadership training and evaluation, judgement and decision making.

Forgey, William. Basic Essentials of Hypothermia, 1992, 72 pages. ICS Books, Merrillville, IN

A look at the differences between acute and chronic hypothermia with an emphasis on prevention, diagnosis, and field treatment.

Forgey, William Ed. *Position Papers of the Wilderness Medical Society*, 1994, The Wilderness Medical Society, Indianapolis, IN

Peer reviewed statements concerning pre-hospital care of persons with various injuries sustained in remote areas.

Forgey, William. *Travelers' Medical Resource*, 1991, 892 pages, ICS Books, Merrillville, IN

A thorough look at all aspects of preparing for overseas travel, including disease prevention and an extensive database of disease risk tables by country. Immunizations, insurance, embassy locations for US and Canadian representatives, techniques of minimizing personal danger, and post trip considerations for medical care are all included. This book is perpetually updated with a computerized database which can be contacted by book owners so that the information on disease risk will not become outdated.

Gill, Paul G. *Pocket Guide to Wilderness Medicine*, 1991, 204 pages. Simon & Schuster, New York, NY

This is an excellent book of practical advice that covers both basic and advanced care principles of wilderness related trauma and environmental injuries.

Hodgson, Michael. *The Basic Essentials of Minimizing Impact on the Wilderness*, 1991, 72 pages. ICS Books, Merrillville, IN

This book distinguishes between universal considerations and special rules of minimal impact camping for different ecological zones and helps the reader understand the consequences of the various activities involved in wilderness use.

Houston, Charles S. *High Altitude Illness and Wellness*, 1993, 80 pages. ICS Books, Merrillville, IN

A thorough look at the high altitude illnesses, stressing prevention, diagnosis, and treatment. This book emphasizes the physics and physiology of the normal subject and describes what goes wrong in the abnormal. This is a must have book for anyone planning a trip to high altitudes.

IAMAT, Information Packet, 1994.

Detailed information on prevention, risks, and locations of diseases of importance to travelers, including a list of physicians around the world available to treat IAMAT

members. Information and membership is free, but a voluntary donation is appreciated. In the U.S. contact IAMAT at 417 Center Street, Lewiston, NY 14092 (716) 754-4883 or in Canada at 1287 St. Clair Avenue West, Toronto, Ontario M6E 1B8 (416) 652-0137.

Jacobson, Cliff *Canoeing and Camping: Beyond the Basics,* 1992, 196 pages. ICS Books, Merrillville, IN

This is only one of many skill books which Cliff has written for ICS Books. This includes an overview and advanced techniques of the most important subjects.

Jacobson, Cliff *Canoeing Wild Rivers,* 1989, 355 pages. ICS Books, Merrillville, IN

While designed for remote area canoeing, this book has many valuable tips for any expedition. Advanced map reading and land navigation, concise recommendations concerning camping equipment and technique, and plenty of advice to ensure a successful expedition.

Petzoldt, Paul K. *The New Wilderness Handbook,* 1987, 250 pages. W W Norton Company

This is an update of Paul's original work that describes critical expedition skills such as a proper time plan which takes into consideration geography, people, climate—and this is only part of the expedition planning and execution techniques covered.

Poltano, Colleen *Lost in the Woods—Child Survival for Parents and Teachers,* 1993, 64 pages. ICS Books, Merrillville, IN

Starting with a story to capture children's attention, the book acts as a model of what a well-informed, resourceful child can do when they become lost. The last portion of the book is a series of experiments that a parent or teacher can share with children to teach the basics involved with survival.

Schimelpfenig, Todd, and Linda Linsey, *NOLS Wilderness First Aid,* 2nd Ed, 1991, 356 pages. Stackpole Books, Harrisburg, PA

This is an excellent book with emphasis on recognition and stabilization of injuries, evacuation, hygiene, and emergency procedures for outdoor groups.

Scott, David. *Paradise Creek,* 1985, 160 pages. ICS Books, Merrillville, IN

A book full of insight on what a long term experience in remote wilderness can be like. Not a journal style of book, but a series of episodes that illustrate the challenges, life style, and satisfaction that two nineteen year olds gleaned from a year in the Arctic taiga of Manitoba.

Steele, Peter *Far from Help!* 1991, 214 pages. Cloudcap Press, Seattle, WA

A climbing physician of world renown, Dr Steele's book is full of innovative and field expedient techniques for handling problems.

Tilton, Buck. *Backcountry First Aid & Extended Care,* 2nd Ed 1994, 56 pages. ICS Books, Merrillville, IN

A quick reference highlighting the information in Medicine for the Backcountry, this is an excellent small book to carry in the field.

Tilton, Buck and Hubbell, Frank. *Medicine for the Backcountry,* 2nd Ed 1994, 192 pages. ICS Books, Merrillville, IN.

This outstanding book is a must have for any backcountry traveler. It emphasizes assessment, packaging, transport, and reassessment issues. This is the perfect companion piece to my book, Wilderness Medicine.

Wilkerson, James A., Ed. *Medicine for Mountaineering,* 4th Ed 1992, 416 pages. The Mountaineers Books, Seattle, WA.

The distilled knowledge of a large group of physician authors, the depth of technical detail make this an excellent reference book for mountaineering and remote area travel.

Appendix D

FOOTNOTES

1. A discussion of group dynamics is found in the book *Wilderness Educator* by the Wilderness Education Association, listed in Appendix C.

2. The definitive treatise of planning considerations of time, terrain, weather, and group capabilities is found in *The Wilderness Handbook* by Paul Petzoldt, listed in Appendix C.

3. *Medicine for the Backcountry*, 2nd Edition (1994), by BuckTilton and Frank Hubbell, is the best book written concerning patient assessment and stabilization for evacuation. It is available from the publisher, ICS Books, PO Box 10767 Merrillville, IN 46411-0767, Telephone (800) 541-7323, $12.99 plus $1.50 shipping and handling.

4. This section has been adapted with permission from *Medicine for the Backcountry*, by Tilton and Hubbell.

5. The American National Standards Institute, or ANSI, establishes specifications for many manufactured products. For further information on the harmful effects of ultraviolet light obtain a copy of *Ozone, UV and Your Health: 50 Ways to Save Your Skin* (1994), by Buck Tilton and Roger G. Cox, available from ICS Books for $6.99 plus $1.50 shipping and handling. This 55 pagebook reviews all aspects of protection from UV.

6. A comprehensive list of disease risk by country is contained in my book *Travelers' Medical Resource*, 895 pages, available from ICS Books for $19.95 plus $2.50 postage and handling.

7. IAMAT (The International Association of Medical Assistance for Travelers) can be contacted at 417 Center Street, Lewiston, NY 14092; telephone (716) 754-4883. Please send a voluntary contribution to cover the cost of any salt packets which you request, at least 25 cents each, plus shipping cost.

8. *The Basic Essentials of Minimizing Impact on the Wilderness,*by Michael Hodgson, is available from the Publisher, ICS Books,for $5.99.

9. Howell, JM and Stair, TO: Topical Antibiotics for All Wounds? *Annals of Emergency Medicine.* 1992; 140:1516.

[10.] This section has been included from *Medicine for the Backcountry*, by Tilton and Hubbell.

[11.] Chan D., Goldberg R, Tascone A, Harmon S, Chan L: The effect of spinal immobilization on healthy volunteers. Ann EmergMed. January 1994; 23:48-51.

[12.] A complete list of country risk factors is contained in mybook, *Travelers' Medical Resource*, listed above.

[13.] CDC. Rabies Prevention - United States, 1991. *MMWR*; RR-3:5.

[14.] Crouse JC, Josephs D., Health Care Needs of Appalachian TrailHikers. *The Journal of Family Medicine* 1993; 36:521-525.

[15.] The reader is referred to Dr Forgey's book, *The Basic Essentials of Hypothermia,* ICS Books, 1991, for a full discussion of the physiological changes of rapid onset and delayed onsethypothermia, including prevention, diagnosis, and treatment (see Appendix C).

[16.] There is a distinct difference between immersion and submersion. Submersion indicates that the victim is entirely under water; immersion means that the head is above water.

[17.] The reader is also referred to a recent, excellent book by Charles S. Houston, M.D., *High Altitude: Illness and Wellness,* ICS Books, 1993, for $6.99 plus $1.50 postage and handling (800)541- 7323.

CLINICAL REFERENCE INDEX